Menopause

Menopause

HELP AND HOPE FOR THIS PASSAGE

SALLY CONWAY

PYRANEE
BOOKS

Zondervan Publishing House
Grand Rapids, Michigan

MENOPAUSE
Copyright © 1990 by Sally Conway

A Pyranee Book
Published by Zondervan Publishing House,
1415 Lake Drive SE, Grand Rapids, MI 49506.

Library of Congress Cataloging-in-Publication Data

Conway, Sally
    Menopause: help and hope for this passage / Sally Conway.
        p. cm.
    Includes bibliographical references.
    ISBN 0-310-52271-4
    1. Menopause. 2. Middle-aged women—Religious life. I. Title.
BV4527C6559   1990
618.1'75—dc20   89–29635
                                                                   CIP

Printed in the United States of America

90 91 92 93 94 95 96 / PP / 10 9 8 7 6 5 4 3 2 1

THIS BOOK IS DEDICATED WITH
OVERFLOWING LOVE
TO THE SPECIAL WOMEN IN MY LIFE:

MY DEAR MOTHER,
Altha Larson Christon

MY WONDERFUL DAUGHTERS,
Barbara Schneider
Brenda Russell
Becki Sanders

MY PRECIOUS GRANDDAUGHTER,
Hayden Anne Sanders
and any other granddaughters yet to come

Contents

PART III

SURVIVING AND THRIVING

Acknowledgments

I am indebted to a number of people who have unselfishly given of their time and expertise to help this book come to fruition:

My husband, Jim, who was my greatest encourager, insight-giver, and housekeeper during this season of re-searching and writing the book.

My three daughters—Barbara, Brenda, and Becki—who have taught me much about being a woman and have also encouraged me to write this book.

My Menopause Support Group—Anne Sanders, Carol Bridgeford, Mary Turner, and Marilyn Jordan—who have truly supported me, prayed for me, and kept me inspired. Special thanks go to Marilyn, who is also an assistant at Mid-Life Dimensions, a registered nurse and one of my medical advisors, and a hands-on aide to me.

My Care Group—Jacque Coulombe and Karen Dirks—who have nourished me, kept me accountable, and cared that I got this book written.

Ruth Dix, M.D. *and J. Bruce Cox*, M.D., two gynecologists who carefully read and corrected the manuscript to ensure accuracy. Another family practice physician also gave invaluable counsel, but he does not wish to be named.

The researchers and writers whose material I gleaned and distilled to pass on to my readers. I have tried carefully to give credit where credit is due.

The 436 women who responded to my National Study of Menopause Survey and the many other women who have shared their menopausal histories with me.

My secretaries—Susan Hall, Sally Pede, and Karen Mattox—who capably handled office details so I was free to work.

My editor—Sandra Vander Zicht—and all the other editors, assistants, and publishers at Zondervan who have worked to bring this book to completion.

And, finally, *you*, dear reader, for having courage to get help by reading *Menopause: Help and Hope for This Passage*.

Important Note to Reader

This book is intended to provide general information about menopause; it is NOT a substitute for professional care. Each woman's situation is unique, and new research continues to expand medical knowledge, so consult a physician for help with individual symptoms.

The author and publisher have made every effort to ensure that medical information is accurate and in accordance with accepted standards at the time of publication. The reader, however, is advised to consult a reputable, caring professional and to follow the product information sheet included with any prescribed drugs. This book is provided to help you select the best professional help and be informed about available options for health care.

In some instances, names and exact circumstances have been changed to protect the privacy of individuals.

PART I

ENCOUNTER
WITH MENOPAUSE

1
You Are Here

Marjorie was a woman you would have liked for a friend. She had everything: a loving family, a good job, numerous friends, and a strong faith. She was warm, caring, intelligent, loved her husband and children, and had a sparkle about her. Marjorie worked as a nursing supervisor in a well-respected hospital in a midwestern city. She faithfully attended church and a weekly Bible study. She delighted in having people in her home and made her guests feel special.

But Marjorie was experiencing menopause, and it was overwhelming her. She had seen two or three doctors. They were slow to help. Her husband was understanding—to a point.

Her friends were never much help. The ones in the Bible study group assured her that she just needed to pray more intensely. Her pastor's wife, a kindly older woman, told her she wouldn't have any trouble if she would just trust and obey God.

Marjorie became more and more depressed. Her husband was having a harder time understanding her; her friends made her feel guilty. Her doctors didn't take the opportunity to help her fast enough.

Majorie's body chemistry became so unbalanced from a rapid decrease in estrogen that she had little emotional strength left. After more than two years of struggling to get herself under control, she could try no longer. For days she frantically—and unsuccessfully—reached out for understanding from her husband and friends. She called her doctor one morning with another plea for some relief. He implied her problems were mostly her imagination.

Marjorie hung up the phone, walked to the garage, and, without opening the garage door, started her car. Her husband came home that evening and found his lovely Christian wife dead.

HELP!

Admittedly, Marjorie's case is extreme. But many menopausal women suffer needlessly for years. They are not getting the help they need to live most successfully through this time. They are a pain to those around them and *in* pain themselves. Not only are they miserable now, but worse, they may be setting themselves up for future problems.

Perhaps at some time you have been in a huge, unfamiliar shopping mall. You wanted to get to a certain store you knew was in the mall, but you couldn't find it. What's more, in the labyrinth of oddly shaped wings lined with shops, you didn't even know where you were.

How glad you were to find the large directory of stores! First, you looked for the highlighted spot that boldly proclaimed, "You are here." Aha! Now you had a start on getting where you wanted to go.

This chapter is designed to help you get your bearings. Then you may more easily get where you want to go as you find your way through this unknown menopause time.

My own interest in menopause began around age 40 when I realized that someday it would happen to me. I wanted to be as well informed as possible. I was already bleeding heavily when I had my period, experiencing drastic mood swings, and having occasional hot flashes. So I went to my gynecologist and asked if I could be starting menopause. He said I was too young.

When I told him that my moods were up and down— uncharacteristic of my previous experience—he immediately suggested that I see the psychiatrist in his medical group. He went on to imply, rather directly, that my troubles were all in my head.

On my next visit, to care for some follow-up matters, I again asked for information about menopause. His waiting room and patient rooms had several little display boxes about family planning, natural childbirth, breastfeeding, and other materials for young, childbearing women. No literature was available for older women's concerns. When I pressed him, he said, "Well, there's something around here somewhere," and went off. In about 10 minutes, he returned with a battered little booklet, which he gave to me.

I was unaware that with every Pap smear he took, he received a lab report of my estrogen level that would have given some indication of a menopausal condition. He didn't tell me and I didn't know enough to ask for the results.

After two or three years, the hot flashes stopped and my moods leveled out again. On one of my later visits to him, I mentioned that my earlier spells had stopped. He said haughtily, "Well, since you're still menstruating, it's obvious that it wasn't menopause, isn't it?"

WHAT LIES AHEAD

What I know now—and what is only beginning to be told to us—is that our ovarian function begins to fluctuate around age 35. Some of us experience "menopausal" symptoms years before the actual menopause occurs. It would help women in their late 30s and early 40s to know this fact and to know what can be done about it.

When menopause does occur, many women suffer needlessly from hot flashes, vaginal and urinary problems, aches and pains, tingly skin, strange emotions, and exaggerated feelings. We think we should be strong enough to manage this physical passage of life without trauma. If we are depressed, angry, nervous, or easily rattled, we may feel we've become weak, so we add *guilt* to our other problems.

Relationship complications at this time in life may also add to our difficulties. Most women's feeling of well-being is greatly influenced by what is happening with the people who mean the most to them. Children are growing up and going away, parents are getting older and needier, husbands may be facing drastic work dilemmas or wanting out of the marriage. Or there may be no husband and no children—and many regrets about that.

In any case, menopause may seem like one more of life's cruelties. At best, we feel it's sort of a vague, unknown wilderness for which we have no map. We know we have to walk through it, but we are afraid of the pits in which we might get mired and don't know how to skirt the thick forests with the bears we've heard about.

MY INTEREST

My own menopause was sudden and final: I had a "complete" hysterectomy at age 50. Even though I thought I was well-informed, I'm now surprised at how little I knew. I had asked the doctors my questions, but wasn't aware of how much there was to know! And they didn't volunteer any extra information.

Because of the work my husband and I do with mid-life men and women through our organization, Mid-Life Dimensions,[1] I have talked one-on-one with hundreds of menopausal women. Many have very sad stories. They have been misunderstood by their families and belittled by their doctors. Worst of all, they have mistreated themselves. My personal friends and relatives were also reporting similar experiences.

The more I listened and observed, the more I was convinced that we women at this age need to take responsibility for ourselves. We can become better informed about the latest medical facts, find a doctor who will be of genuine help, learn the right questions to ask, and help our families and co-workers understand this special time in our lives. We must be aware of our physical symptoms and honest about our emotions.

After my hysterectomy, I began to study menopause more intensely than before. I read the latest research, got special permission to attend an eight-hour medical seminar, and interviewed doctors. Using a six-page questionnaire, I also conducted a national survey of 436 women. (A sample of this questionnaire is at the back of the book.)

In addition, I invited women who are going through what I am to attend a Menopause Support Group. This ongoing relationship is a wonderful learning arena. More than just gleaning facts for a book, I'm continuing to profit personally from the strength and insight of these women. We are friends who love each other.

WE'RE IN THIS TOGETHER

I'd like to share with you what I've learned. I want to help you help yourself. You may feel like you don't know where to start. You may think you don't have time to take care of your needs. You may feel too weak or confused. Or you may be saying, "What's the big deal, anyway? Menopause is a natural thing. I'll get through it."

Yes, menopause is natural. So is childbirth. So is death. But all hurt. These "natural" events affect some people more than others. The good news is that help is available.

Forty million women in the United States are currently of menopausal age. How many have a difficult time? No one knows for sure. Researchers' reports of women vary with each study. Some authorities state that at least 75 percent to 80 percent of menopausal women experience moderate to severe hot flashes, sleeplessness, strange skin sensations, mood swings, and heart palpitations.[2]

My survey of 436 women revealed that 70 percent had most of the usual physical problems: hot flashes, vaginal dryness, urinary incontinence, painful joints, sleep problems, and heart palpitations. Hot flashes were reported by 87 percent of the women; more than 81 percent had sleep problems.

The number of women who suffer *emotional* problems because of hormone imbalance at menopause is even more difficult to determine. Does menopause actually affect emotions? Or does an emotional state affect menopause?

Some researchers boldly proclaim, "Family troubles, not the climacteric [the time around menopause], cause midlife blues."[3] Or, "The majority of menopausal women report no depression."[4] However, other experts feel that many previously stable women have great difficulty managing ordinary life stresses until their bodies adapt to the drastic decline in estrogen.[5]

Again, my study revealed that 72 percent of the women were experiencing emotional responses noticeably stronger than previous patterns. These included such symptoms as depression, anger, anxiety, impatience, low self-esteem, and a fatalistic view of life. More than 37 percent of the women reported having thoughts of suicide! Over 85 percent had an increase in nervousness, irritability, and forgetfulness.

BOUNCING OFF THE WALLS

Actually, an individual woman may not care much about the statistics, other than to know she's not alone in this crazy battle. What she cares about is how *she* is feeling.

How does she cope with her hot flashes? Why is she so unusually tired? What is this creepy, itchy feeling all over her body? Why is sex so painful? What should she do about the times when her heart seems to race or skip a beat? Will she ever get a decent night's sleep again? Why won't her doctor help?

And where did this anger and rage come from? One moment she's never felt so upset in her life. The next moment she's laughing giddily. It seems good just to act silly. Oops! Suddenly she feels sad and blue. She starts crying and can't stop.

A few hours later she feels euphoric and sublimely happy. The world looks so wonderful and she loves everybody. She wants to throw up her arms and sing joyously. Oh! Oh! Something her husband just said sounds fishy. He *has* been acting strangely. She wonders if he's having an affair. How terrible! How could he do this? Oh, the awful ache in the pit of her stomach! How will she ever make it? But then maybe she's just imagining her husband's unfaithfulness.

This zigzag of emotions is wearing her out! Physical problems mixed with tiring mood swings and questionable perceptions about everything drain her energy and motivation. She decides she must be going crazy.

THE "BEST" IS YET TO COME?

Worse than the immediate misery are the future problems. Right now, I'm not talking about what she *fears* may happen—whether her husband will be faithful, her grown children love her, or society respect her as an older woman. I'm referring to the changes in her body because of menopause that will affect the rest of her life.

It's not merely that she's no longer menstruating, but other very concrete, scientifically observable changes are taking place in her body that will affect the quality and quantity of her life. Aging occurs for both men and women, but changes in a menopausal woman's body are much more drastic. Menopause means she now lacks the estrogen that is vital to the functioning and health of many of her body systems.

She needs to know that her bones are at high risk for osteoporosis and that the possibility of heart attack or other serious cardiovascular problems is much greater than before menopause. Her sexual activity could be affected because her vaginal area will undergo great changes. She also may have continual urinary infections or incontinence.

But, she needs to know the good news! For the most part, all these consequences can be prevented or greatly lessened. As dire as all the possibilities are, we live at a wonderful time. New discoveries for our health and well-being are constantly being made.

HOPE AND HELP ARE ON THE WAY

I'm excited about what lies ahead in this book. I'll be expanding on the ideas and facts that I've briefly mentioned in this chapter. Together we'll dig into some medical information, but not so much that it overwhelms you. If you'd like to study in more depth, see the *notes* at the back of the book. A *glossary* of words and terms is also included after the notes.

I'll present menopause realistically, so those of you who are having difficulty can identify with what I'm saying. (I personally have been turned off by books or articles with a Pollyanna approach.) On the other hand, I don't want to get bogged down with a negative attitude, because there's much to be positive about.

Those of you who are fortunate to have had an easy time during menopause may be less inclined to read this, but it contains much crucial information for you too, especially about your future health. Those of you having a horrible time are desperate for some empathy and immediate answers. You've got my ear and my understanding, and I'll try to point you toward help.

I'll talk about what you can do now to make your passage more comfortable and what you need to do for your long-range health. I'll give you hints about how to choose the right doctor and how to ask the right questions. I also want to help you come to terms with your inner self during this very important era of your life.

This book also aims to help your husband and older children understand you. The last chapter is written specifically for them.

Reading this book may also help counselors better understand the physical and psychological elements of this developmental stage of life.

All of us, of every age and stage, need to be good stewards of our bodies, our minds, our psyches, and our relationships. These are God's precious gifts to us. For the menopausal woman, there is no better time than now to begin—or to continue—maximizing her full capacities in every area of life.

I can hear you groaning, "Maximize? I doubt if I can even survive!" This book is for you.

2
First-Time Changes for You

Menopause itself isn't so bad, but its side effects can drive you crazy. You probably don't mind the cessation of menstruation, and you may be very happy not to have to worry about getting pregnant. But the agonies blot out the blessings.

Your mother may have told you there'd be a time like this—but you didn't believe her! Now nobody believes *you*, either. At least, not many. The rest think it's all in your head, you just want sympathy, or you're nothing but a crabby old shrew.

You probably wonder about yourself too. Much of the time you aren't sure who or what you are. You're confused because you're living in an enlightened age when people are expected to understand themselves—emotionally, spiritually, physically, socially, and every other "ally" there is.

You're supposed to be mature. If you're experiencing menopause, you *are* mature—physically. In fact, some would view you as overripe. Your kids think you're old. The younger people you work with, or serve on committees with, or buy cosmetics from, think you're old.

OVER THE HILL?

Most books and magazine articles about menopause, on the other hand, tell you this is a wonderful age. The prime of life, they call it. They declare that you're on the edge of a new beginning. You feel "on the edge" all right—on the edge and about to go over.

No wonder you're confused. You aren't as antiquated as young people view you, especially in light of the 30 to 40 years you may yet live. Why, those kids haven't even been alive as long as you still have to go! But neither do you feel as full of bliss about the future—or the present, for that matter—as the joy-promoters in those books and articles or on those TV talk shows.

At least, you aren't alone. As I've said, over 40 million women in America are postmenopausal.[1] Since post-menopausal symptoms last from one to 10 years or more, and premenopausal symptoms begin some years before the actual cessation of menstruation, a large number of women are in the throes of the "change of life."

That term, "change of life," makes me grimace. It conjures up childhood memories of old women (at least, they seemed old to me) whispering and knowingly shaking their heads (gray heads, of course). They were discussing some woman not present in the group. This woman was doing strange things and driving everybody else crazy. The gray-haired women would wisely pronounce a diagnosis: "She's going through *the change*."

This time of life *is* life-changing, but so are a lot of other stages of life. The difference now is that many of the changes are irreversible. Some of the changes are great and wonderful! Some are terrible. They force you to search for the "true you"—that beautiful person who must be in there somewhere under all the disintegrating pieces.

Carolyn would understand you. She felt absolutely miserable. And alone. She had been in such terrible agony the last two years that she was ready to give up. She had tried doctors, positive thinking, prayer, exercises at the health club, talking to her Bible study friends, a Caribbean cruise with her husband. Nothing worked.

Nothing relieved her terrible depression and perpetual fatigue. She found little help for the constant aches in her bones and muscles. She couldn't understand why she often felt like crying for no reason.

She and her husband had argued more in the last year than in all their marriage. A few times Dick had become so frustrated, he had yelled and called her "an old bitch." Carolyn had never heard him use that word before and certainly not on her!

Many times in the last several months her teenage daughters had scolded, "Mom, you're so unreasonable! You'd better get some pills or something."

"I'm not being cross," she thought. "Besides, sometimes they deserve it."

She wasn't sleeping well at night and occasionally she felt so hot all over she wondered if she were having hot flashes. She thought she might be starting menopause. She would be 48 soon.

GET BUSY

When she saw her family doctor, he dismissed her symptoms with a wave of his hand, "That's what a woman your age can expect." When she complained about her awful depression, he said it was because she didn't want to see her daughters grow up and the older one leave for college. She just needed to get busy with some interests other than her children.

Yes, Carolyn was interested in her daughters and their activities. She felt that most of the time she and her two girls had a close, fun relationship. She also liked caring for her house and being a companion and lover to her husband. But she was much more than a wife, mother, and housekeeper.

Carolyn was a musician. Her college degree was in music and she was the organist for her church. They had several choirs and she accompanied most of them. That meant many hours of weekly practice, and she thrived on it. Until recently. Now even her music wasn't satisfying.

Carolyn and her family lived in a moderately large midwestern city with several cultural and civic opportunities. Through her church, Carolyn had become involved in a city-wide crisis pregnancy center as a volunteer counselor for a few hours each month. She was also a team leader for her weekly Bible study, and she and her husband entertained many friends in their home.

Lately, however, everything seemed so fruitless and shallow. What did all of this activity mean anyway? She was tired. She just wanted time to herself. But when she did get some free time, she didn't like being alone either.

SAME SONG, SECOND VERSE

She tried a different doctor. But he wasn't keeping up on the current information about treating menopausal symptoms. When she pressed him for a test to measure her estrogen level, he told her that she'd have to go through menopause sooner or later and knowing about her estrogen level wasn't going to change anything. He was still relying on the medical information from the '70s, which had concluded that estrogen therapy for menopausal women increased their risk of cancer. He prescribed an anti-depressant pill instead.

Carolyn tried the pills for a few weeks but was concerned that she might become addicted. She didn't see much difference in her emotions anyway. She quit taking the pills and continued to struggle alone with her symptoms. Some months her period didn't come; when it did, she bled heavily. Worse than this, though, was the awful battle she was having with depression and anger.

Sometimes she tried to talk with other women her age or older about what she was feeling, but they acted like she was strange. Her mother said she hadn't had any trouble with menopause. This wasn't the way Carolyn remembered it, but she didn't press. Maybe her perceptions had been off even when she was younger. The way everything around her was going, she wasn't sure she was seeing *anything* correctly. She felt she was losing her mind.

Carolyn was an intelligent woman, however, and she wasn't a quitter. She also had a warm, personal relationship with Christ and had experienced his help all her adult life. She realized she needed to use all the resources available to her. Besides spending more time praying and reading, she also went to see a third doctor. This took some courage; she was beginning to feel like a hypochondriac.

The new doctor tested her estrogen level and confirmed that menopause was close. However, he did not want to prescribe estrogen therapy at this time. His manner was brusque and Carolyn felt uncomfortable with him.

More months passed and Carolyn went through more emotional and physical misery. She tried another doctor. Starting up with new doctors was beginning to cost a lot of money, but if she could just get some help, it would be worth it. Help had to be out there somewhere.

FAMILIAR REFRAIN

Perhaps Carolyn's story sounds like yours. You could add variations to the same themes of baffling changes in your body and emotions and the often-frustrating search for someone to understand and help you.

The great majority of women in my study had trouble getting information about what was happening to them. One wrote:

My gynecologist, a nice Christian man, had no interest. His only solution was valium and vaginal creams that did not help. I went to another gynecologist. He told me hormones would probably clear up 90 percent of my problems, but he would not prescribe them until I saw a psychiatrist, which I did. But when the psychiatrist wanted to put me on drugs, I quit going to him and went back to my medical doctor, who gave me hormones (without testing).

I cannot believe that a lot of doctors are *still* uninformed or do not believe menopause is a serious problem to be dealt with.

Hundreds of women who answered my survey said they didn't know what was happening to them and kept blaming themselves for not maintaining a good attitude or for acting selfish. Many were not sure if their symptoms warranted seeing a doctor or if they should just tough it out.

In the remainder of this chapter we will touch on some of the significant symptoms and events that may be happening to you at this age. Some of them are more complicated than others and we'll look at them in additional detail in succeeding chapters.

DEFINITIONS

Let's begin by defining certain words we'll be using. The precise definition for *menopause* is the specific point in time when the last menstrual period of your life occurs. But the more common use of the word includes the time span before and after the stopping of menstruation. *Climacteric* is the correct medical term for the period before and after the exact time of the menopause.

In this book we will use the word *menopause* to mean the entire range of time around the specific incident of *the menopause*. It will include premenopausal and postmenopausal symptoms. When we use *the* in front of *menopause—the menopause*—we will be referring to the exact point in time that menstruation stopped.

Remember to refer to the *glossary* at the end of the book when you come to words you don't know. If you know their meanings, you'll be better prepared to talk to your doctor and enlist his or her cooperation in your health care.

IRREGULAR PERIODS

The first symptoms you may notice before the menopause are changes in your menstrual period. You may have an increase in the blood flow or in the number of days your period lasts. Or your blood flow may decrease and your period may skip some months entirely. Your periods may be closer together or farther apart than normal. Doctors call this dysfunctional uterine bleeding.

It is important to keep a calendar, marking the beginning and end of each period and noting the intensity. After a few months, it is easy to forget details, to generalize, or to overemphasize a particular symptom. With a written record, you have more accurate information to share with your doctor.

Abnormal flow or a change in the frequency of your periods should prompt you to see a doctor. Heavy bleeding, for example, may mean *endometrial hyperplasia*, a build up of the lining of your uterus. A possible precursor to a cancerous condition, this should be diagnosed and treated immediately. Let me stress that hemorrhaging does not automatically mean you have cancer. But your doctor needs to monitor your condition, so that you both know whether or not you have a malignancy. The likelihood of cure is very high when treated early.

FIBROID TUMORS

Sometime after age 35, during a pelvic exam by your doctor, you may be told that you have fibroid tumors in your uterus. These tumors are very common: Some estimates are that 30 to 40 percent of all women have them.[2] They are benign and usually small and insignificant. Insignificant, that is, unless they are *your* tumors!

I remember the time when I was on my back on the doctor's table in that graceful position—knees bent, feet in cold stirrups, a paper sheet draped over my legs to provide a false sense of modesty. As he poked and prodded, my gynecologist said, "Hmmmm. Your uterus is about the size of a 12-week pregnancy." After my heart missed a few beats, he added, "It's probably because of fibroid tumors."

"Tumors! Those are something other people have," I thought.

He went on to explain that rarely are such tumors malignant. They can be easily monitored by a periodic exam. They become most bothersome when they cause pain and heavy bleeding during menstruation.

"Well, those are two of the reasons I'm here today," I said.

He went on to say that if they grew to be larger than a three- or four-month pregnancy, he would probably recommend their removal. At his suggestion, since it wasn't a life-threatening condition, I agreed to wait a few months to see what developed.

Removal of fibroid tumors is usually done by hysterectomy, although a procedure known as myomectomy can be performed if a woman still wants to bear children. In a myomectomy the surgeon removes the tumors, leaving the uterus intact. Unfortunately, the tumors may grow back.

If you have been told you have fibroid tumors, you may decide to wait to have them removed if they are not causing undue pain and bleeding. Fibroid tumors are fed by estrogen, and after the menopause, the tumors may shrink and cause no more problems unless you are on an estrogen replacement program.

If you are living with fibroid tumors, your doctor should specify how soon he wishes to check them again. Normally they should be checked every six months.

HOT FLASHES

As menopause advanced for me, I would often wake suddenly at night, feeling as if I were going to burst into flames. I wasn't really sweating as some women do, but I was so terribly hot I couldn't stand it. First I'd peel off the sheets and blanket. Then I'd strip out of my nightgown. I'd turn my pillow over to the cool side. Finally I'd just have to get up and walk around to let the mattress cool down. All this time my husband would be snoring soundly on his side of the bed! I still have the same experience if my estrogen replacement is insufficient.

Other women describe their hot flashes as a time of profuse sweating or "the sweats." They may soak their clothes or bed many times in 24 hours. Sometimes the symptoms are called "hot flushes" because the rise in temperature seems to just flush over the body and then disappear.

One time, as a gentle, older usher at our church took hold of my arm to help me to a seat, he sighed softly, "Oh, oh! You're glowing. I remember when my wife used to do that." Even though I was a little embarrassed, I thought "glowing" was a nice way to put it.

Women in the professional world are often ashamed to have anyone know they are suffering from hot flashes. It really isn't too dignified to be giving a business report or teaching a class with perspiration running down your face and arms. What's worse is to be standing there also wondering if your sanitary napkin is going to hold the flood of blood you feel gushing out of your body.

Women are many times subjected to humiliating situations because of their bodies! But perhaps we can learn to meet these times with a touch of humor, some preparedness, and some openness with others so that we don't feel persecuted. God has not made a mistake. And he's not picking on women.

It's better to be able to talk about hot flashes when it's appropriate. Joke a little. Let those closest to you know when you are physically uncomfortable. Ask them to cooperate by arranging a cooler setting for you. We will talk more about hot flashes and relief from them in Chapters 5 and 6.

ACHES, PAINS, AND OTHER INDIGNITIES

Another first for you as you encounter menopause may be unusual aches and pains in your joints and muscles. Many women have had some of this before now, but the pain may increase greatly during menopause.

Or you may have strange tingling sensations on your skin. Some women feel as though ants are crawling over them. Others report a burning sensation.

One morning I awoke, certain that water was trickling from the top of my head, over my left temple, and down my cheek. When I reached to wipe it away, I found nothing.

In a few hours the sensation changed to a general tingling feeling in various parts of my face. As the days wore on, I had other strange prickles and tingles running around my body. I reported this to my family doctor who sent me to a neurologist. After some preliminary testing, the specialist said the results were inconclusive. If it were something serious like multiple sclerosis or a brain tumor, it would have to develop further to be diagnosed. Since I was going to be moving in a few months, the doctor and I decided I should wait and find a new doctor if the symptoms persisted when I got to California.

In our new home the tingling feelings increased and became very distracting to my concentration. I complained to two gynecologists and three family practice doctors. Then I saw another neurologist. After some initial tests, but without going the ultimate route of CAT scans and other more expensive procedures, this specialist said that I would just have to "live with it."

I now know that decreasing estrogen can cause tingling, prickling sensations.[3] Lack of estrogen also causes an increase in joint and muscle pain.[4] However, these symptoms can also be caused by other serious problems, and it is wise to tell your physician what you are experiencing. But do remind him or her of your age and your estrogen decline!

You may also experience more vaginal and urinary discomfort now. Infections might be more frequent, vaginal dryness may be a problem, and sexual intercourse may be painful. Again, the dwindling supply of estrogen is probably the culprit. Chapters 5 and 6 will help you decide what to do to manage these situations.

ROLLER-COASTER FEELINGS

In addition to your physical body giving you problems, you may find your moods going up and down, in and out. This is normal. But normal doesn't mean comfortable, does it?

You will want to find help to get stabilized, but knowing that many other women go through the same emotional upheavals is some consolation. Many women don't understand what is happening and berate themselves for being weak.

A 42-year-old midwestern woman wrote, "At times I feel like I'm going under. Everything seems like it is on fast forward and out of control. I feel panicky and think that I'm accomplishing nothing even though I manage a department [at work] and have five children."

A lovely, gracious school teacher in my Menopause Support Group said recently, "I kept blaming myself for not being in better control. My doctor was a wonderful help and assured me that it wasn't my fault. He prescribed estrogen and I couldn't believe the difference in only two weeks!"

Many women's self-esteem takes a beating at this time. They feel rejected, suspicious, and overly critical. They may be "picky, picky" about little details, and then feel unable to make ordinary decisions. Routine tasks seem insurmountable. Some women are acutely sensitive to noise, temperature, and people's offhand remarks. They have trouble concentrating.

About four years ago I jotted a brief, disjointed note in my journal:

> Lack of concentration/short attention span. Thoughts come and go; jump in and out. Seem urgent at the time; then quickly forget. Remember again. And seem urgent once more.

A little later I wrote in the same journal about myself:

> Paranoia—uncertain and then certain about particular fears and suspicions. Then uncertain again.

No wonder we menopausal women question our sanity! These feelings and behaviors are so much more exaggerated than ever before in our lives—we are truly puzzled.

CHANGING ROLES

Added to our physical discomforts and psychological dilemmas is the fact that our job description is changing. Menopause generally takes place at the time when women who are mothers are finding themselves running out of a job—the job that for so many years seemed like a lifetime occupation.

As they learn to relate to their grown, or almost-grown children, even women who have a good peer relationship with their children often wonder where the boundaries are. At a time when her self-esteem is so precarious, a menopausal woman feels she is in quicksand. She wants to relate to her adult children in a way that respects their autonomy, but she often questions where her own selfhood comes into the picture.

The women in my Menopause Support Group often express concerns about their roles with their grown children. One day a usually very self-assured professional woman said, with a tremble in her voice, "I feel very vulnerable to my family right now. When I was a young mother, I was much more certain about my role. I was sure about my decisions. Everything was so much more concrete then. Now I just never know for sure ... "

JUST THE TWO OF YOU AGAIN

Even women who feel very comfortable with most aspects of their empty nest say that the restructuring of their marriage relationship can be tricky. Yes, it can be an exciting adventure if you and your husband are happy together. But even then, the game needs new rules. The number of players is the same as it was when you started marriage but your years of life experience make for new dynamics.

One woman in my study explained, "My husband and I both began our changes at the same time without being aware of each other's problems . . . Our most difficult time in life was compounded by each of us needing help all at once. No one was there to put a Band-Aid on the wounds fast enough to hold the marriage life's blood in."

A wife may be displaced by divorce or, at least, her husband's preoccupation with his last mad dash to make it in his career. Or he could be wrestling with his own mid-life reevaluation and be oblivious to his wife and her needs.[5] A single woman who has always wanted to be married may be in agony as she comes to menopause and feels cheated out of the opportunity to have children. Even the intentionally single woman may have second thoughts about her decision to concentrate on her career in place of having a family.

ADAPT, ADAPT, ADAPT!

Working women, whether married or single, may find their roles changing on the job as expectations shift. This may be a fun challenge or it may seem too demanding. Work colleagues may accept and appreciate her for her wisdom, or they may feel she's outdated. For one reason or another, she may be faced with leaving her job. The adjustment could be overwhelming.

Aging parents also become more predominant in our lives about now. While we were busy keeping up with our children, meeting our husband's needs, running a household, and perhaps holding down a job, we let our parents live their own lives. And, generally, they were able to. Now they have needs that we must help meet.

We are in strange territory. We are not accustomed to making decisions *for* our parents. In fact, we still may be trying to prove our maturity so that they'll quit making decisions for *us*. Now, however, because of declining health and resources, our parents or our husband's parents may need emotional, financial, and face-to-face help from us.

Usually they aren't emotionally ready for our help either. Or they let us take over in one area at one time, but at another time or in another area, they may be fiercely independent. It's a hard time of life for them too. As my 82-year-old mother says, "I've never been old before." In all of the changes, we need to help our parents keep their dignity.

Then our siblings and other friends add to the mix of all the roles to which we are adapting. You've noticed, haven't you, that life is made up of a series of transition times and crises? Your sister may be starting menopause, your brother wrestling with mid-life crisis, your neighbor getting divorced, your boss facing retirement, and your best friend moving across the continent. Most women have known—mentally—that some of these changes were coming when they actually arrive, but owning the emerging new roles is more difficult.[6]

MOUNTAINS AND MOLEHILLS

Somehow we were better able to keep up with changes before menopause hit. Strong women start coming apart and struggle with everyday stresses.

Is it simply mind over matter? Are we just not accepting our changing situation? Or could it be that a hormonal imbalance is altering our perception?

Now that Premenstrual Syndrome (PMS) has been getting the recognition it deserves, women in menopause can hope for more understanding. Medical scientists and the general public have come to acknowledge that the body's chemical balance has a great deal to do with our psychological well-being.

A woman in her late 20s, who knows I am working on this book, said to me the other day, "I can understand how a lack of estrogen could affect a menopausal woman's emotions. For two days this week I was fighting with my husband, angry at everybody else, and feeling like all the world was unfair. Then my period came yesterday. Sure enough, this morning my world looks like a wonderful place to be. My circumstances are the same, but they look so much different than they did earlier this week."

Postmenopausal women whose emotions get back under control, either through replacement therapy or the natural adaptation of their bodies, say that their domain returns to normal. That's encouraging for the woman who is still in the pits, bouncing this way and that, and wondering if life will always be that way. Carolyn, the musician who was in terrible agony for two years, finally found the help she needed from a fourth doctor. She was relieved to know her symptoms actually were because of hormone fluctuations and she could get stabilized by taking progesterone prescribed by her doctor. As her life greatly improved, she wondered why it had been so hard to get the information she needed.

Many women have expressed to me, in personal conversations and on the questionnaires, that menopause is just not discussed very much. It's hard to get facts. One 52-year-old nurse wrote, "No one talks about it. No one shares any personal information about it. I feel so alone—as if I'm the only woman going through this bewildering period of life."

Well, she's not alone. You aren't either. If there are 40 million of us, with 3,500 women a day joining our group, we belong to a big clan. Let's learn all we can about menopause and our future health. Let's begin to discuss the topic, so that we're better able to deal with this sometimes traumatic transition.

3
Our Foremothers

We are probably going to live at least a third of our life after menopause. According to most statistics, the average age for menopause is 51.5. A baby girl born in America today can expect to live to age 79.5.[1]

The more years you live, the more you can expect to live—up to a point. If you have reached age 50 in good health, some statisticians say you can expect to live to age 92.[2] Others say you'll live only 30 or 35 years more. Either way, that's a lot of life left to live!

This morning as I struggled to get my back, feet, and legs working when I got out of bed and limped toward the bathroom, I thought to myself, "Oh, well, I should expect these joints to be uncooperative after all these years. They eventually get going every day, so I'll manage. I can just plan

45

to be a little crippled a couple of hours each morning for the rest of my life."

"For the rest of my life!" I suddenly yelled inside. I just realized that could be another 30 or 40 years. Do I want to put up with the pain and inconvenience of rebellious joints for that long?

The same goes for my attitudes and my relationships. Do I want to just let them coast? While my husband, Jim, and I were celebrating our 35th wedding anniversary with an exhilarating trip to Hawaii, I said many times, "Just think, we may have another 35 years together!" Every time I said that, I nudged myself a little, asking what I was doing to build for a happy 35 more years.

FROM HERE TO ETERNITY

When we realize we have so many years left to live, we may have to make some adjustments. We might need to set goals we want to reach, make plans for continued growth, cultivate relationships, and work on some of our nastier personality traits. We aren't just going to rock away in our secure little corner by the fireplace for five more years and then be gone.

At the turn of the century many women never reached menopause. Their average life expectancy was 48 years. The ones still alive probably had children at home during menopause because they gave birth to more children and at a later age than today's women. They didn't have to worry about what to do with themselves after their children left home. Their health was such that they were expected to act like "old ladies."

Of course, we're speaking "on the average" and "statistically." You may have had a great, great grandmother who lived to be 90, but this was the exception. You may know someone today who just had a baby at age 48, but again, that's a rarity. The average woman in generally good health today can expect to live 30 to 35 years after her children leave and after her ovaries cease to produce estrogen. In succeeding chapters we will discuss in detail what estrogen does for the health of many body parts—bones, vasomotor system, skin, cardiovascular system, and vagina, to name a few.

We will also see how lack of estrogen can cause a number of problems for our future health:

- weak bones that fracture easily and cause us to be stooped
- heart attacks, strokes, and other cardiovascular problems
- faster aging in our vaginal and urinary areas, which can mean painful sex and more infections
- older looking skin

And, of course, we can't overlook the *immediate* discomforts of the menopausal period: hot flashes, increased aches and pains, fatigue and malaise, memory lapses, depression, and scrambled emotions.

HAS SOMEONE GOOFED?

Human females are the only mammals who continue to live long after their ovaries cease to function. Some medical scientists have raised the question of whether it's some kind of a mistake that women now live so many years without estrogen.

These new developments may have caught humanity offguard, but God's not surprised. Our Creator knew all along what we women would be experiencing in the 20th and 21st centuries. In addition, the wisdom for saving and prolonging life came from him. He is the source of the skills, machines, methods, and medicines from which we now profit.

So we live longer and do so without our body's natural estrogen. Our responsibility is to make the best use of current knowledge and apply it toward caring for the life God has given us. We owe it to ourselves, to those around us, and to the One who created us. You could call it "stewardship of the temple."

IN THE GOOD OLD DAYS

We can be thankful that we live now rather than a few generations ago when menopause was very "hush-hush." Then, women usually didn't discuss the matter among themselves, with their families, or with doctors. Propriety dictated that they keep female health problems quiet. If they consulted a doctor, he generally was at a loss for effective treatment because of inadequate medical knowledge.

A hundred years ago most women's health was fragile by age 40, and menopause greatly compounded existing problems. Ignorance and inappropriate modesty killed many of our great, great grandmothers and kept their sisters in needlessly poor health.

A study of medical literature available in the mid-1800s reveals much. Dr. Charles Meigs, in his book, *Woman: Her Diseases and Remedies, Letters to His Class*, explains why treatment was so difficult:

> The relations between the sexes are of so delicate a character, that the duties of a medical practitioner are necessarily more difficult, when he comes to take charge of a patient laboring under any one of the great host of female complaints. . . . So great, indeed, is the embarrassment arising from fastidiousness on the part either of the female herself, or of the practitioner, or both, that, I am persuaded, much of the ill success of treatment may be justly charged thereto.

Dr. Meigs then reveals a startling viewpoint:

> I confess I am proud to say that, in this country generally . . . women prefer to suffer the extremity of danger and pain rather than waive those scruples of delicacy which prevent their maladies from being fully explored. I think this is an evidence of the presence of a fine morality in our society.

Whoa, there, Dr. Meigs! So that's what happened to my female ancestors. Now I know why the tombstones in those fascinating old cemeteries show that so many women died too young. Well, to give Dr. Meigs proper credit, he does go on to say,

> It is true that a greater candor on the part of the patient, and a more resolute and careful inquiry on that of the practitioner, would scarcely fail to bring to light, in

their early stages, the curable maladies, which, by faults on
both sides, are now misunderstood, because concealed,
and consequently, mismanaged and rendered at last
incurable.

Even though Dr. Meigs felt a need for "greater candor,"
he did not approve of newspaper advertisements that
showed women wearing "utero-abdominal supporters" and
other such devices. I can almost hear him hissing and huffing
as he asked, "Who wants to know, or who ought to know that
the ladies have abdomens and wombs but us doctors? When
I was young, a woman had no legs even, but only feet, and
possibly *ankles*; now, forsooth, they have utero-abdominal
supporters, not in fact only, but in the very newspapers."[3]
I'm just glad that I'm alive now and that I can claim my
body parts unashamedly. If I need help to keep them all
going in the same direction, I can get that help. I may have to
persist and insist, but help is available.

MORE OF THE GOOD OLD DAYS

We can understand why 19th-century women were afraid
of doctors. Catharine Beecher, author of *Letters to the People on
Health and Happiness*, attempted to alert her readers to the
terrible suffering women experienced with doctors. She
herself was inhibited in the language she used, so we can
only imagine exact details:

> During the later periods of my investigations in regard
> to health, I became aware, not only of the general decay of
> the health of my own sex, but of the terrible suffering, both
> physical and mental, produced by internal organic dis-

placements, resulting chiefly from a general debility of constitution. . . .

She went on to say that in many cases "there was no possible remedy for this appalling evil but daily *mechanical operations, both external and internal.*" And since these "operations" were mainly "performed with bolted doors and curtained windows, and with no one present but patient and operator, there was a painful apprehension of evils."[4]

One of America's first female doctors, Elizabeth Blackwell, who practiced medicine in the latter half of the 19th century, wrote, "The *standard of health* among American women is so low that few have a correct idea of *what a healthy woman is.*"[5] Twenty years later a professor of medicine at Harvard College noted, "The delicate bloom, early but rapidly fading beauty, and singular pallor of American girls and women have almost passed into proverb. The first observation of a European that lands upon our shores is that our women are a feeble race."[6]

Feeble race, of course! Our foremothers worked long hours with no labor-saving appliances. They gave birth to many children under hazardous conditions. The infant mortality rate was high, and diseases like pneumonia, smallpox, and flu took high tolls on the health and life of people of all ages.

If women lived through these ordeals to experience menopause, they suffered alone or endured a doctor's bizarre treatments. Hot flashes were relieved by extracting blood, either with leeches or by "cupping," a procedure in which glass cups were heated and applied to the skin to draw the blood to or through the surface. Many women feared that the end of menstruation allowed poisons to build up in the body, but Dr. Edward Dixon in *Woman and Her Diseases* explained that the end of the menses "must probably be the cause of considerable derangement in the circulation" and that the affliction could be alleviated by "drawing a small quantity of blood from the arm."

Excessive menstrual bleeding was treated with cold packs on the lower abdomen while the rest of the body was kept warm. If a woman fainted, Dr. Dixon recommended that a person of "clear judgment and a cool head" give the woman a tablespoon of brandy and water every 10 or 15 minutes until the doctor arrived.[7]

Purges of Epsom salts or castor oil "to cool the system" during a woman's "critical period" or douches with "cold slippery-elm water five or six times a day" were some of the suggested treatments.[8]

Women were absolutely to refrain from sleeping on a feather bed, which could "promote plethoric accumulations, uterine hemorrhage, and constipation of the bowels." Worst of all, it might "excite the generative organs, which should henceforth be left, as far as possible, in a state of inaction. [A woman at this age should] avoid all such circumstances as might tend to awaken any erotic thoughts in the mind, and reanimate a sentiment that ought rather to become extinct, such as the spectacle of lascivious figures, the reading of passionate novels, and . . . every thing calculated to cause regret for charms that are lost, and enjoyments that are ended for ever."[9] (I hope you are looking forward to Chapter 8—our discussion of sex for today's woman!)

HERE COMES LYDIA!

Because of the deficiency of medical advice, women turned to home remedies and tonics such as Lydia E. Pinkham's Vegetable Compound. You have perhaps seen the reproductions of ads for her product on wallpaper and restaurant table tops featuring old-time newspaper decor. I am old enough to remember seeing the actual advertisements and the bottles in my grandmothers' medicine cabinets.

Lydia Pinkham was targeting menopausal women with her ads:

> There is no period in a woman's career which she approaches with so much anxiety as the "change of life." It is surprising what happy changes LYDIA E. PINKHAM'S VEGETABLE COMPOUND brings about in this condition. So marked is its power that all the trying days of the Change may be passed over in perfect safety. Women who have been dreading the Change, who have been taught to look upon it as something horrible, may now lay all such anxiety aside. Thousands of letters from women tell me that their life of distress and sleeplessness was changed to one of perfect comfort almost immediately.[10]

Some of the advertisements featured pictures of women endorsing the health tonic. One was the county president of the Women's Christian Temperance Union (WCTU) of Kansas City:

> Give Mrs. Pinkham a chance—I know she can help you as she did me. The world praises great reformers. . . . Among them all Lydia E. Pinkham's name goes to posterity

with a softly breathed blessing from the lips of thousands upon thousands of women who have been restored to their families when life hung by a thread, and by thousands of others whose weary, aching limbs [she has] quickened and whose pains [she has] taken away.[11]

Another endorsement came from the treasurer of the Kansas City WCTU:

> My dear sisters: I believe in advocating and upholding everything that will lift up and help women, and but little use appears all knowledge and learning if you have not the health to enjoy it.
>
> Having found by personal experience that Lydia E. Pinkham's Vegetable Compound is a medicine of rare virtue, and having seen dozens of cures where my suffering sisters have been dragged back to life and usefulness from an untimely grave simply by the use of a few bottles of that Compound, I must proclaim its virtues, or I should not be doing my duty to suffering mothers and dragged-out housekeepers.
>
> Dear Sister, is your health poor, do you feel worn out and used up, especially do you have any of the troubles which beset our sex, take my advice; let the doctors alone, try Lydia E. Pinkham's Vegetable Compound; it is better than any and all doctors, for it *cures*, and *they do not*.[12]

It's amusing to me that the compound so readily endorsed by these women of the temperance union contained 18 percent alcohol!

We enlightened women of this decade might scoff at the use of such a medicine, but government tests conducted in the 1940s proved that Lydia Pinkham may have been ahead of her time. In addition to its calming properties, the tonic was found to reduce hot flashes and to correct menstrual irregularities.

The tests showed that Lydia Pinkham's formula contained "hormonal factors," and "estrogenic materials, or principles capable of being converted into estrogen by chemical means." These apparently came from some of the plants used. Lydia Pinkham had openly advertised that her compound was made of "true unicorn root, false unicorn root, life root, black cohosh, pleurisy root, and fenugreek seed."[13]

To me, using Lydia E. Pinkham's Vegetable Compound for menopausal symptoms doesn't sound any crazier than sucking blood out of women by leeches or warm cups. In fact, it was probably much better because of the estrogenic materials.

WHOM CAN WE COPY?

Our ancestors looked for relief from the agonies of menopause, but in a sense we are the inexperienced pioneers on the frontier of long life after menopause. Until recently, we have had very few role models of older, vigorous, healthy women. The two generations before our mothers had some elderly women, but not many of them could be called active and healthy after age 70.

Even in this decade I have been with groups of women in their 40s and 50s who are looking forward to dawdling away the rest of their years. They feel it's their due. "After all," they say, "I've had a lifetime of hard work and pressure."

What a waste! Take a group of 20 women who each have

at least 30 more healthy years to live, and that's 600 years thrown away. These women generally have not had examples of older women who lived a vigorous life and made a difference in the world.

I am more often with women who are aware they still have productive years ahead, but they aren't sure how to best use them or how to find the health to enjoy them. Many women are at a loss about what steps to take for a meaningful life after their children have left home. They may enjoy homemaking—up to a point. After all these years, however, they realize that a house can take every bit of time they give it and it's never enough. They ask, "Do I want to get to eternity and say to God, 'I spent the last 30 years keeping a clean, well-decorated house, Lord'?"

Some women *may* spend their last 30 years keeping an immaculate house, but the happiest ones do it with specific goals in mind. They view their home as a haven for the tired and hurting. They may provide a place for youth gatherings, a young moms' monthly meeting, or various support groups.

Most married women today, however, find that they must help with the income for a number of years. Single women work outside of the home out of necessity. Other women have careers or do volunteer work just because they want to or because they feel called to share their abilities and talents.

Chapter 14 contains some ideas on how to make your years count for the most. Call this the "stewardship of time."

FROM FERTILITY TO FUTILITY?

Menopausal women may decide, intellectually, how they will care for their bodies and make the best use of their time, but often their emotions aren't in tune with their best intentions. Menopause, after all, really does cause tremendous modifications in our lives. That's why—even though I shudder at the term—it is appropriately called "the change of life."

We go from being women capable of childbearing to women who are no longer fertile. Even if we never intend to produce another baby, we may grieve over not being able to. We like to feel that we have the power to choose.

Down through the centuries—in legend, literature, and Scripture—the admired and sought after woman was the one who could bear children. Other qualities—unselfish spirit, vivacious personality, endless energy, and thin, firm body, to name a few—are considered attractive today. But many of these desirable traits come automatically by being young.

Our culture has put such a high premium on youthfulness that menopausal women get hit with a double whammy. Not only do they struggle with the actual physical discomforts of the climacteric, but they also face disdain—or at best, indifference—because they are no longer young.

In addition to moving from fertility to infertility and from being young to being old, we also shift from being actively needed as a mother to possibly being a spasmodic and barely tolerated consultant. We must say good-bye to a very fulfilling era of life, and we may not be ready to greet the new stage.

Yes, I acknowledge again that our personal attitudes about our attractiveness and place on earth have much to do with our happiness and how others perceive us. But many previously happy, self-confident women now find their joy and confidence slipping away during the upheavals of menopause.

ARE WE IN THE RIGHT PLACE?

In some other cultures older women are given a more respected status. Anthropologist Margaret Mead reported that, in Bali, postmenopausal women and virgin girls are permitted in some ceremonies where menstruating women are not. Older women are allowed greater freedom in their speech and behavior.[14]

In China, before the revolution, postmenopausal women, for the first time in their lives, could be free of male domination and even assume domination over men.[15] Other cultures studied by Pauline Bart also provide an improved position for women after menopause.[16]

About now, you may be thinking of the place of older women in Scripture. Titus 2:4-5 specifically gives older women the privilege and responsibility of teaching younger women how to live.

When I was young, I couldn't picture myself ever knowing enough to pass on to anyone else. From my vantage point now, however, I see that I do have insights for the young. Living life and evaluating that life under God's guidance gives women—and men too—a wisdom that comes only with age.

Older American women have value, but it may not always be noticed, especially while they're in the throes of menopause. Women in our culture generally haven't called attention to menopause. The people around them haven't either, other than to poke fun at hot flashes or to complain or get angry about their erratic behavior.

Some women do have supportive husbands, children, and friends. About half of the women in my study said their husbands had been a help. But many said their husbands had been no help or made matters worse.

Children were a help to only 35 percent of the women; mothers were a help to only 12 percent. Over 36 percent of the women noted that a friend or number of friends had been a help.

"DOCTOR, CAN YOU HELP?"

Receiving sympathetic medical help for menopause is also difficult. In my survey only 26 percent of the women reported that their doctors were helpful.

Perhaps this is because, historically, many doctors have paid little attention to menopause. Since it's not a disease (and many women would hasten to add, "since it's not something that happens to men"), little research has been devoted to menopause symptoms until recently.

Dr. Lila Nachtigall, a renowned reproductive endocrinologist, has worked for 20 years in the field of estrogen metabolism and estrogen replacement. Her name kept appearing as I searched for meaningful, accurate, scientific facts on menopause. She says in her helpful book, *Estrogen: The Facts Can Change Your Life*:

Menopause has been neglected because it is strictly a *woman's* problem. Men don't go through menopause—the

idea of a true male menopause is a highly exploited myth.
If men did have a menopause and quit producing
testosterone, the major hormone responsible for their
maleness, is it possible to imagine they would not make
every effort to replace it? If it was shown to be safe, are
there any intelligent men who savor life who wouldn't take
hormone pills?

Besides, virtually all physicians and researchers are
men, the very people who need not be concerned with
menopause and who may indeed feel threatened by it.
Menopause has not been a subject that has warranted
concentrated attention from them. Instead, it has often
been perceived as a rather amusing and trivial problem,
something neurotic women without much else to do made
an inordinate fuss about.

But now, with greater numbers of women entering
medicine and the demands of women to be treated equally
and seriously, plus the more enlightened attitudes of
many male physicians, we're already seeing much more
attention paid to all of the problems that are exclusively
female.[17]

GRADUATION TIME

This "change of life" is difficult, partly because no "rite of
passage" has been accorded menopause as is generally
bestowed on other life-changing events. We have rites of
passage for birth, death, and marriage. We usually have
celebrations or observances for other transition times, too,
such as when we begin and end a job, start college, graduate,
get our driver's license, retire, and even when we move.

Puberty is a recognized transition. As difficult as adoles-
cence may be for everyone involved, it is, at least, a time of

"progress," a time of gain, of hope, of moving forward. Menopause, on the other hand, is more often viewed as a time of loss, of bleakness, of charging downhill at breakneck speed.

The *onset* of menstruation is often celebrated. The girl and her family joyfully recognize that she has entered a new stage of life. Why not honor the *cessation* of menstruation? If menopause could have a noble tradition attached, perhaps it would be easier to take.

People who study rites of passage for various life events generally recognize three stages: "First, isolation or withdrawal from society; then the stage of ordeal, involving physical or symbolic renunciation and confrontation with loss and death; and finally the stage of renewal and rebirth after change."[18] This would seem to be very appropriate for dealing with the transition of menopause.

It would help if we felt we were passing into an era of life with some rights and privileges to compensate for the losses of youth. We could create a rite of passage that would include an appropriate time of grieving, followed by some sort of celebration, and then move on to our new status.

Actually, in many ways we are privileged to be living in a time of increased medical knowledge and a new openness. I personally have seen a great change since the late '70s. Researching this book over a number of years, I have been excited to see the medical community becoming much more involved in studying menopause and in helping women now than it was at the beginning of my study.

Even though we don't have many models to follow as we launch into this long postmenopausal time ahead of us, we have stronger support and more resources than women have ever had. We have the opportunity to expand the awareness that has begun. Perhaps this will even be the generation that creates an honorable rite of passage for menopause.

PART II

OLD WIVES' TALES, NEW WIVES' TALES, AND FACTS

4
Your Wonderful Body

The container you came in—isn't it a marvelous gift? Your body is one of the most priceless treasures you have on earth. It's what holds *you*. Right now, though, you may be thinking that your "crate" is certainly substandard! Your aches and pains, hot flashes, weight problems, urinary infections, and chronic tiredness don't seem like much of a present. You may even be going through the tediousness of fighting a serious disease or recovering from an injury or from surgery. Your body may seem like more of a burden than a blessing.

I can easily identify with you in some of your misery. However, every time I think about all the intricate workings of our physical bodies, I am filled with awe. I don't understand a fraction of what there is to know about how our bodies operate, but what little I do comprehend makes me wonder how they hold together as well as they do. (Especially when we sometimes abuse them so.)

In this chapter we will consider our reproductive system and related areas. I don't intend to give you a boring, hard-to-understand biology lesson; I do hope you will get a better understanding of God's wonderful plan for how the system is supposed to work.

As you read, you may be like I was a few years ago when I first read *No More Hot Flashes and Other Good News* by Penny Wise Budoff and *Change for the Better* by Orene Schoenfeld and Beverly Smith.[1] Even though I didn't grasp everything in those books about how ovaries, glands, hormones, and other mysterious-but-vital parts and pieces function, I was left with a great appreciation for God's blueprint for our menstrual cycle.

SO MANY EGGS, SO LITTLE TIME

The plan begins when we are just a little more than a gleam in our mother's eye. We're a tiny, little being, blissfully nestled away in mommy's warm, nourishing womb, but we already have our own womb, ovaries, and millions of egg cells. (Wow! Aren't we glad those don't all become babies!) What starts out as about 5 million *oocytes* (potential eggs) when we are a 20-week-old fetus is reduced to only 1 or 2 million by the time we are born.[2]

By our early teens, or perhaps as early as 10 years of age, we reach puberty. At puberty the cells surrounding each *ovum* (egg) in our ovaries form a *follicle* and produce the hormones, estrogen and progesterone. Our monthly menstrual cycle has begun. We are "fertile."

At the onset of our first menstrual period, we have only about 300,000 to 400,000 ova remaining in our ovaries. (How would you like to hatch even *this* many babies?) Of course, a part of the plan is that, with the help of a husband, some of those ova *will* develop into children during your years of fertility. Most women, however, use only a few of these eggs in their lifetime. Even if a woman is never impregnated, she is reminded each month when she menstruates that she is capable of reproduction.

By age 40 we are left with a mere 10,000 ova. We actually release only 300 to 400 of those in the entire 35 to 40 years we menstruate. What happens to all those millions of other little ova? They simply atrophy. (The same as some other parts of our body!)

Sometime after age 35 our production of estrogen declines and no more ova are released each month. In the mid- to late 40s, menopause usually starts in earnest. By the early 50s the process that took place at puberty has reversed, menstruation has stopped, and we are infertile for the rest of our lives. Not only are we unable to be pregnant, but without estrogen we are more prone to osteoporosis, heart problems, and complications due to degeneration of the vagina, urinary tract, skin, and other tissues.

"THIS LITTLE THING TOUCHES OFF THESE OTHER LITTLE THINGS"

The monthly menstrual cycle reminds me of a marvelously complex factory or processing plant. If you've ever visited a beverage bottling plant, a meat-packing company, a fruit-packing operation, the packaging section of a bakery, a lumber mill, or an elaborate dairy milking barn, you know what I mean. Someone throws a switch that starts motors, conveyer belts, and all sorts of machines. Things are moving forward, up and down, in and out. Each part of the operation works with all the other parts. The action of one piece triggers another piece. If a problem occurs in one part of the line, it affects the entire operation. The end product is the result of all the parts working together smoothly.

Our monthly period is not just a flow of blood we must care for until it stops. Nor is our monthly cycle only an egg being released from an ovary, traveling through a fallopian tube to the uterus, and—since it was not fertilized by a male sperm—moving along with the unused uterine lining on out through the vagina.

All that's involved in the menstrual cycle is awe-inspiring! But since we're not medical students, we'll only consider its rudimentary elements. This will be enough to help us appreciate the wonderful process that has been going on in our bodies all these years without much effort from us. We have not had to say, "Okay now, hypothalamus, it's time for you to signal my pituitary gland to release the follicle-stimulating hormone."

THE NORMAL CYCLE

The plan—which began when we each received our own little reproductive system at conception and which swings into full action at puberty—is set in motion by the *hypothalamus*. Located in our brain, the hypothalamus is a control center for our glands. It signals our *pituitary gland*, located at the base of our brain just below the hypothalamus, to release FSH (follicle-stimulating hormone). The FSH then travels through our bloodstream to our ovaries in our lower abdomen.

Inside our ovaries are the thousands of ova (eggs), which are contained in little depressions called *follicles*. The FSH lives up to its name (follicle-stimulating hormone) by activating one of the follicles to begin to mature.

THE EGG OF THE MONTH

While the chosen follicle is developing, FSH is also stimulating the ovum in the follicle to mature. At the same time, a thick layer of cells gathers around the follicle and ovum. These cells secrete estrogen in the form of *estradiol*. They also bathe and nourish the ovum. The estradiol circulates in the bloodstream, causing the uterus to develop a soft, rich lining, known as the *endometrium*, in preparation for the arrival of a fertilized egg.

These activities take place in about 14 days, starting with the first day of menstrual flow. This is known as the "estrogen" or "follicular" phase of the menstrual cycle.

"HEY, P.G., GIVE HER ANOTHER JOLT!"

The increased estrogen level in our blood now prompts our hypothalamus to stimulate our pituitary gland to release a greater amount of FSH and a surge of a second hormone, LH, or luteinizing hormone. This rush of LH into the bloodstream causes the developing follicle to enlarge and rupture.

The ovum separates from the follicle and, with its follicular fluid, is propelled through the surface of the ovary. Ovulation has occurred. (All of this takes place in an ovary about the size of a walnut.) The mature ovum is then picked up by the delicate ends of the fallopian tube and moved along to the uterus.

ENTER PROGESTERONE

Meanwhile, back at the site of the ruptured follicle, the follicle becomes a bright yellow spot on the ovary known as the *corpus luteum*. The corpus luteum secretes estrogen and another very crucial hormone, *progesterone*, into the system.

Didn't I tell you this would be fun? Stick with me because these details are the foundation for making wise choices about your future health. I'll be telling you more about the importance of progesterone for postmenopausal women as we go along.

During the menstrual years, progesterone is the controller of the second 14-day stage, the "luteal" phase, of the cycle. Progesterone causes the uterine lining, which started to grow under the influence of the estrogen, to mature further in preparation for a fertilized ovum to become implanted and develop into a fetus (baby).

Progesterone actually stops the effects of estrogen by causing the cells in the uterine lining to quit multiplying and begin maturing to nourish the egg. In addition, progesterone inhibits the hypothalamus from signaling for more FSH, which would start a new cycle.

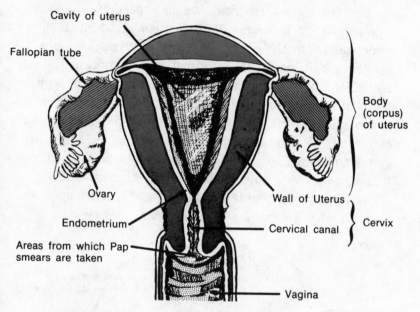

Cavity of uterus

Fallopian tube

Body (corpus) of uterus

Ovary

Wall of Uterus

Endometrium

Cervical canal

Cervix

Areas from which Pap smears are taken

Vagina

FRONT VIEW OF FEMALE INTERNAL ORGANS

If pregnancy does occur, the corpus luteum continues to produce the progesterone necessary to maintain pregnancy for the first 10 weeks after fertilization. After 10 weeks the placenta takes over.

If the egg is not fertilized, LH decreases, the corpus luteum degenerates, and progesterone production falls. As progesterone and estrogen levels drop, the lining breaks away from the uterine wall, and menstruation begins.

The decline of progesterone frees the hypothalamus to signal the pituitary gland to secrete FSH once more. The FSH stimulates the development of another follicle in an ovary. A new cycle has begun.

Isn't this system amazing? We are indeed "fearfully and wonderfully made." Even though medical scientists now understand something about our reproductive system, many mysteries still remain. How does the FSH "decide" which particular follicle and ovum to stimulate each month? Why is the menstrual process so standardized that the normal cycle is generally 28 days? Yes, variations do occur, but given the complexity of all the organs, glands, hormones, and other components involved, it's no wonder that glitches happen, or that some women have a shorter or longer cycle.

Following is a simple diagram I have found helpful to envision what happens during the menstrual cycle.

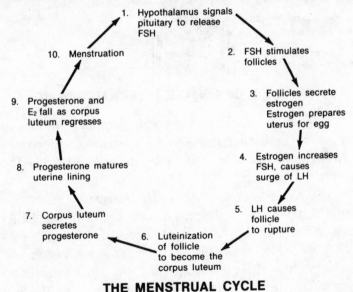

1. Hypothalamus signals pituitary to release FSH

2. FSH stimulates follicles

3. Follicles secrete estrogen
Estrogen prepares uterus for egg

4. Estrogen increases FSH, causes surge of LH

5. LH causes follicle to rupture

6. Luteinization of follicle to become the corpus luteum

7. Corpus luteum secretes progesterone

8. Progesterone matures uterine lining

9. Progesterone and E2 fall as corpus luteum regresses

10. Menstruation

THE MENSTRUAL CYCLE

THEN COMES A CHANGE

Sometime around age 35, the function of our ovaries starts to decline. Our reproductive cycle begins to phase itself out. The number of follicles decreases, and so does the usual amount of estrogen and progesterone that flows back in the blood to shut off the pituitary gland.

When our pituitary gland does not receive enough estrogen and progesterone, it pumps more FSH and LH into the bloodstream to try to spur the ovaries into action. As the ovaries continue to fail, the FSH level keeps rising, sometimes as much as 13 times higher than normal. The LH level may increase three times the usual amount. (A blood test to check our FSH level helps our doctor know if we are nearing menopause.)

These changes in estrogen and progesterone levels affect the phases of our cycle and, thus, the regularity of menstruation. Ovulation may still occur. In time, however, the follicles stop maturing fully and no progesterone is produced.

Without progesterone, estrogen causes the uterine lining to grow unchecked. As the lining continues to increase, it outgrows its blood supply and begins a haphazard disintegration. The menstrual flow is heavy, sporadic, and long. Some women, on the other hand, have a low level of estrogen along with a low level of progesterone. This may cause prolonged, but scant spotting. Eventually, for all women, estrogen produced by the follicles decreases to such a low level that the uterine lining no longer grows. Menopause has occurred.

BUT WATCH OUT!

On our own, we won't know definitely that the menopause has happened. Even after we have missed a period for several months, a belated egg may be released. It is possible for that one egg to be fertilized and become a "menopause baby"! To avoid an unplanned pregnancy, we need contraceptive methods for 12 months after the last period.

A baby now not only would greatly alter our lifestyle, drain our rapidly waning energy, and commit us to a direct mothering role until our 70s, but the child would less likely be healthy. The closer we are to menopause when we conceive, the greater our baby's chances for birth defects. (One out of 32 babies born to mothers at age 45 have Down's Syndrome. By age 49 the incidence rises to one out of 12.[3]) Also, the older we are, the more liable we are to have a spontaneous miscarriage with all its side effects to our own health and emotions.

I once had a dear little student whom the other teachers called "her mother's change-of-life baby." Julie was seeing me for remedial reading, not because she wasn't intelligent, but because her many physical problems had caused her to miss a great deal of school.

She had undergone numerous surgeries to correct missing or deformed areas of her body. Thin and frail, Julie walked with the aid of braces and caught every infection that blew through the school. Because of her braces and lack of stamina, she was unable to take part in physical education class or to run and play during recess.

She wore a hearing aid and had trouble speaking understandably. Initially, she had to work to win the friendship of new schoolmates. She was a plucky little gal, though, and people liked her once they could understand her speech.

Few would say she shouldn't have been born, but as a child Julie endured so much pain, and now as an adult, she faces an every day struggle with her many disabilities.

FOR SURE

Once 12 months have passed after our last period, we may assume we have truly experienced the menopause. However, we no longer have to wait a year to know for sure, since it's possible to have a blood test to measure our FSH level. This test will indicate immediately if menopause has occurred. A blood test to measure estrogen or a Pap smear maturation index can be used to determine hormone function, although neither of these is as accurate as an FSH analysis.

Once we know for sure that menopause has happened, we may celebrate—or go into mourning—or both. We are no longer fertile and, therefore, can no longer become pregnant.

ALL IS NOT TOTALLY QUIET
ON THE HOME FRONT

Even after our ovaries no longer produce estrogen after the menopause, our body does still produce a very small amount of estrogen in the form of estradiol, estrone, and estriol. Estrone is mainly produced in body fat cells. Estriol is made from estrone. In fact, the more fat cells we have, the

more estrogenic substances our body makes after menopause.

"Good news!" you say. Almost. If it weren't for a 400 to
500 percent greater risk of uterine cancer, plus other cancers
and heart disease, chubby postmenopausal women would be
healthier than skinny ones. Fatter women often have an
easier time during menopause, but the continued estrogen
exposure without the counterbalance of progesterone after
menopause does increase the danger of cancer in heavy
women who still have their uterus. All of the sources I
researched, however, maintained that it is healthier to be a
little plump than to be thin after menopause—as long as we
aren't obese.[4] Most of us are going to be sure to remember
that fact and use it when need!

Even though a little estrogen is still being produced after
menopause, it is almost insignificant for most of us. One
needs much more estrogen to prevent damage from the host
of possible marauders. Just as a reminder, some of them are:

- osteoporosis
- heart disease
- hot flashes
- vaginal dryness and atrophy
- urinary infections and incontinence
- insomnia
- tingling skin
- nervousness, depression, anxiety, forgetfulness.

MENOPAUSE OUT OF SYNC

The degree of agony is usually even worse for women
who experience an early menopause because of surgical

removal of their ovaries or because of destruction of their ovaries by radiation or chemotherapy. Apparently, the sudden withdrawal of estrogen causes menopausal symptoms to be more severe. The body has not had time to gradually adjust to the loss. The extraglandular sites for converting precursor hormones to estrogen have not yet gone into business.

Women who have an early natural menopause don't seem to experience the symptoms so severely. Scientists think perhaps this is because the body has had fewer years to depend on estrogen. The loss doesn't come as such a jolt.

Menopause is considered premature if it comes before age 35.[5] Early menopause may be hereditary, or it may be caused by diseases such as lupus, multiple sclerosis, or even arthritis. Premature menopause may also occur because of abnormal chromosomes that limited the number of follicles and ova a girl had during her prenatal formation. When the supply of ova are gone, menopause occurs. Early menopause affects about 8 percent of women.

The women in my study who had an early menopause, naturally or surgically, talked often about the isolation and misunderstandings they experienced. No one their age could identify with them. Older women didn't either. Sometimes their own mothers hadn't yet had menopause. Some still wanted more children. They were angry about aging so early.

One wrote,

Daily, I watch deep lines form under my eyes. Dark circles and puffiness last all day. I feel very old and look even worse. I feel very embarrassed about the whole process. My hair is mostly gray and none of my friends have even a fleck.

At least, menopause will be over someday, and then when all my friends are grumpy (with their menopause), I'll have bundles of energy—I hope.

Menopausal symptoms that begin after age 35 are considered to be the normal slowing of ovarian function that eventually leads to menopause. A woman may begin to notice hot flashes and other symptoms while she continues to have periods. She should consult her doctor about whether to use an estrogen supplement while still menstruating. To help decide, an FSH analysis should be done by way of a blood test. A doctor also may prescribe progesterone to control early symptoms. Women who are under the care of a concerned doctor in the years prior to menopause can avoid most of the awful symptoms.

About 5 percent of women have a belated menopause after age 55. Late menopause is usually a blessing in disguise. These women will more likely retain a youthful appearance longer, their bladder and vagina will not atrophy so soon, they will be less prone to heart attacks and stroke, and they will delay their risk of osteoporosis. Women with a delayed menopause, however, will have continued menstrual periods and chance of pregnancy, along with a slightly increased risk of ovarian cancer. If they are faithful in having an annual checkup with a pelvic examination, however, the threat will be reduced, and they will have had the great benefits of their own estrogen longer.

By the way, women who smoke will probably experience menopause five to 10 years earlier than women who don't.

That means more years for osteoporosis, heart attacks, strokes, and other long-term problems to have a whack at their body.[6] Many physicians stress that smoking is the greatest health hazard anyone can experience.

NEXT ACT!

When we were young girls just beginning to menstruate, we had no idea what life held in store for us. We didn't know if we would have children or how many we would have. We couldn't have known if our menstrual cycle would be interrupted by illness or injury. And we certainly didn't think much about our own menopause!

Now we are faced with the end of our menstrual cycle. Whether we have an early spontaneous menopause, an induced menopause, a late menopause, or an on-time menopause, we can't ignore that we're at the conclusion of our fertility. Our infertility may make us glad, sad, or mad, but we can't escape the other consequences of the cessation of our menstrual cycle.

This is one of those times when "to be forewarned is to be forearmed." You may be learning about menopause ahead of time, right in the middle, or a little late, but there's no better time than *now* to discover what you can do for your own health when your reproductive years are over.

5
Now That Reproduction Is Over

"Menopause is awful! Nothing about your body is the same."

"I just want to scream and run away. I hate myself. I can't get anything done and I'm overwhelmed. I'm tired all the time no matter how much sleep I get or how well I eat or what my blood count is."

"It's scary. I'm not in control of my body. I don't know what's normal or not normal. I'm afraid to see a doctor."

"I can't function normally. I can't make decisions—all projects seem like *big ones*—I lack incentive to complete or even start projects—even housecleaning is now a 'project.'"

"I don't even know myself anymore. I'm not the same person I used to be."

These are only a few remarks from the women in my study. I could give you 400 more, but you get the picture.

Menopause is the time for:
Degeneration
Decline
Depression
Deprivation
Deterioration

Cheery news, isn't it? Especially when we realize that the *de-* prefix means "to reverse or "undo."

However, menopause can also mean:
Renewal
Regeneration
Release
Restoration
Re-creation

Even though we prefer to "accentuate the positive and eliminate the negative," we first need to look at the downside of menopause. Knowledge of what to expect can help us prevent, or at least minimize, the adverse effects.

VASOMOTOR SYMPTOMS

Hot flashes, nervousness, heart palpitations, tingly skin, insomnia, and dizziness—all these at menopause are most likely caused by a vasomotor system dysfunction (there's another of those *d* words).

To understand what *vasomotor* means, it helps to break the word down into its two parts: *vaso* (blood vessel), and *motor* (movement). Thus, *vasomotor* literally means "blood vessel movement."

The vasomotor nerves control the enlarging and shrinking of our blood vessels. These nerves receive cues from our body temperature. If we're cold, the vessels contract and draw blood deep inside the body to conserve heat. If we're warm, the vessels expand, allowing the blood to ventilate. Our hormones help transmit messages to the nerves. When our hormones become erratic, the signals to the vasomotor nerves are not reliable.

I've often told Jim that I seem to have a a malfunctioning thermostat. When I start to get warm, the thermostat doesn't shut off until I'm extremely hot. And when I get cold, it takes forever for it to kick in and warm me up.

Hot flashes (or "flushes" or "the sweats") are part of this problem. So are tingling skin, irritability, nervousness, and jumpiness. The vasomotor nerves are getting the wrong signals or getting them at the wrong times. Dizziness and heart palpitations also can be caused by disruption in blood flow.

SO NOW WHAT?

Hormone replacement therapy often takes care of these symptoms immediately. However, we shouldn't assume that estrogen deprivation is always the reason for dizziness, palpitations, or the other problems. We should mention them to our doctor so that he or she can eliminate other causes.

If we cannot use estrogen replacement (because of estrogen-dependent cancer or other rare reasons), our doctor can prescribe alternate remedies such as progesterone without estrogen, tranquilizers, or medicines such as Bellergal or Clonidine. But these treatments can have serious side effects, especially if we have certain other health problems, and they will not protect against osteoporosis, cardiovascular problems, or vaginal atrophy.

Some women believe that vitamin B, C, and/or E supplements ease hot flashes and other vasomotor symptoms. Not much medical proof exists to substantiate this, but some doctors do recommend these particular vitamins for other health needs, which we'll mention as we go along. Dr. Lila Nachtigall suggests the use of 800 to 1,600 units of vitamin E daily to relieve hot flashes and other vasomotor symptoms.[1] Some doctors, however, warn that high dosages of vitamin E may be toxic.

Occasionally, doctors recommend the use of vitamin B^{12}, vitamin B^6, or lecithin supplements for depression or memory loss that may accompany menopause. I suggest you see a doctor who is trained in nutrition to give you the right guidance.

Other women use herbal teas to relieve menopausal symptoms. It *is* a good idea to reduce caffeine intake, so substituting herbal teas in moderation for coffee can be helpful. Most medical people won't recommend herbal products in place of standard treatment, however, because of the lack of scientific evaluation of herbs and the danger of overdosing on them. In fact, physicians warn against ginseng tea, in particular. Ginseng is a potent source of estrogen, and, in tea, it's very difficult to regulate the amount taken in. Without progesterone to oppose the estrogen, excessive amounts of uterine lining may build up and hyperplasia (a possible pre-cancer stage) may develop.

Whether or not we take anything for hot flashes, we can relieve some discomfort by wearing cool clothing. We should choose short sleeves and cotton. We can wear layers of clothing so that we can peel or add as necessary. Since stress seems to help precipitate hot flashes, we should try to remain emotionally "cool" too.

Ultimately, time will help our vasomotor symptoms. I can hear you saying, "Sure, given enough time, I'll die. Then I won't have any menopausal symptoms!" What I mean, though, is that even without estrogen replacement, our vasomotor system will eventually stabilize. The timing differs for different women, but gradually the vasomotor nerves adjust to the absence of estrogen.

THE AGONY AND THE ATROPHY

Some conditions will *never* be relieved without estrogen; they will only get worse. We don't notice these things at first because they usually come on gradually. The truth is, though, they start advancing as soon as estrogen retreats.

Our skin, membranes, and other tissues begin to dry up. Wrinkles think it's time for a free-for-all! The layers of tissue just under the skin go into default and start making us look like little old dried-apple ladies. We can try to beat this game by gaining weight, but what kind of victory is that? We *still* have wrinkles and our double chins simply look like double chins on old women.

The only thing thin about us is our hair. And it's probably dry and scruffy, as are the cuticles around our fingernails. Speaking of fingernails, they have changed too; they peel and break or have ridges. When we study our hands, we're shocked: they're beginning to look like our grandmothers' hands. They are wrinkled and leathery, and the blood veins and old age spots compete for prominence.

The skin and membranes of women who smoke or who have had a great deal of sun exposure will be worse. Collagen in the skin is depleted by both nicotine and sun.

Men, of course, wrinkle too, but generally not nearly as severely or as early as women.

INNER BEAUTY?

Besides our obvious outer deterioration, inner changes also take place. In our vagina, the membranes dry and the walls thin and lose elasticity. We may find intercourse painful and almost impossible. Due to the discomfort, our sexual desire will likely go on a spiraling decline. Even without pain, our sex drive or libido may dwindle due to the lack of estrogen.

Because the distance between the vagina and the urethra becomes shorter, vaginal and urinary infections occur more easily. The vaginal and urethral tissues get thinner and more delicate. Burning, itching, and irritation are frequent.

Adding to our fun may be involuntary wetting when we sneeze, cough, laugh, or jump. This is usually caused by relaxed pelvic muscles and connective tissues, and a tired-out bladder sphincter.

Grim, isn't it? If you're reading this book late at night, you probably can hardly wait to go on. Your elation over such good news will arouse you so much you won't be able to sleep.

Well, I'm sorry to have to tell you this, but the insomnia you're experiencing is most likely also caused by lack of estrogen. So is the unusual fatigue you've been feeling, as well as the unbearable aches and pains in your bones, joints, and muscles.

UNBELIEVABLE!

The few women who don't experience these symptoms at menopause are going to think we're making up all these afflictions. So are the men. But take hope. Positive shifts in attitudes are taking place. In the years since I began studying menopause, many more doctors and researchers have turned their attention to these symptoms and are finding that they are often caused by the hormonal changes at menopause. They are also working on ways to help.

I'd be glad if they found a cure for the easy weight gain and unflattering body shape changes that occur after menopause. Even with the same amount of food and exercise as before menopause, we gain weight more easily after menopause. Some of it, of course, is because our metabolism slows. If we're on estrogen replacement, we may also find it harder to keep off extra weight.

How our weight is distributed also changes. Our waist, shoulders, and upper back often get more fat tissue while hips and breasts lose some. That means we look more like a cereal box than an hour glass! If we develop osteoporosis and get a dowager's hump on our back, we are a cereal box with a lump.

SO WHAT ARE WE TO DO?

Some postmenopausal changes can't be reversed; others can, and still others can be slowed. Creams and lotions will moisturize dry skin, but—in spite of advertisers' claims— they won't restore the diminishing tissues underneath the skin. Facelifts help for a time, but they are expensive and don't last. This is not to rule out moisturizers and facelifts; we just need to know how much to expect from them.

I suggest that you get good counsel if you're considering cosmetic surgery. Get two or more opinions from doctors who don't know each other. Talk to people who have had such surgery. The public library has up-to-date books that explain cosmetic surgery in lay language.

Keeping skin softened with lotions and moisturizers will help minimize wrinkles. I personally use three or four times more lotions and creams than I did a few years ago. At first, I thought I shouldn't spend the money. Then I decided that if a doctor had prescribed them to combat the dryness that was irritating me, I'd buy them. So why not do it at my own direction? My skin feels more comfortable, and it looks better, even if I don't look 30 anymore.

Estrogen is the best help for keeping skin and membranes moist. If you have a problem with vaginal dryness during intercourse and are not using estrogen replacement, or you need help in addition to estrogen, lubricating jelly can be purchased without a prescription and will help with dryness. Use a water-soluble jelly rather than a petroleum-based one. Several brands are available on the shelf with feminine hygiene products. Vaginal suppositories to aid lubrication are also available.

Estrogen cream, which is applied vaginally, is often prescribed to combat dryness. Within a few days it restores natural lubrication and thickens the vaginal walls so that the end result is even better than lubricating jelly. New over-the-counter, but non-estrogenic products that help thicken vaginal walls are now available also. These are particularly good for the woman who shouldn't have estrogen.

SOME MORE WORDS TO THE WISE

If you have minor vaginal irritation or burning, you may find that nonprescription topical creams and ointments will give relief. But yeast or bacterial infections or sexually transmitted diseases need a doctor's help. This is also true if you have a bladder infection.

After menopause the bladder and urinary tract become more alkaline than acidic. Since acid fights harmful bacteria and other organisms, postmenopausal women are more susceptible to infections. Here are some hints to help prevent urinary infections:

- Wipe from front to back after urinating so that germs from your rectum are not brought forward to your vagina and urethra.
- Urinate within 10 minutes before and after sexual intercourse.

- Urinate frequently throughout the day rather than keep your bladder full for hours.
- Drink eight to 10 glasses of water a day so that your urine is less concentrated and is not providing a fertile breeding ground for infectious organisms.
- Drink cranberry juice for prevention as well as for clearing up an infection. It provides an acidic urinary tract and bladder similar to premenopausal conditions. The recommended amount is eight to 16 ounces spaced throughout the day.
- Take large doses of vitamin C (as much as 1000 mg a day) which also provides acid.
- Eat yogurt containing live culture. This will increase the desirable lactobacilli in the vagina.[2]

TINKLE, TINKLE

For the problem of incontinence (involuntary urinating), you may find some help before you have to give in to buying adult diapers or protective pads. Even if you have to wear diapers, it's no longer a horrible stigma. In the last few months, I've seen several advertisements and coupons for different brands of adult diapers. (So far, I haven't saved any of the coupons!)

Bladder corrective surgery is one option for help with your unexpected wetting. Again, you'll want at least two medical opinions. Some women are glad they have had it; many others say the pain was not worth the benefit that lasted only a few years. Some women absolutely must have the surgery because of the serious prolapse of their bladder.

Another help for bladder control, as well as for toning up the vagina, is to do Kegel exercises. You can do these easy exercises wherever you are and as often as you think of it. The goal is to tighten the bladder sphincter and pelvic floor muscles around the urethra and vagina. To do this, contract your muscles as if you were stopping yourself while urinating. The pattern is to contract, hold a few seconds, release. Repeat for 10 to 25 times each session and try to do a few sessions every day.

These exercises can be done as you sit at your desk, stand at the kitchen sink, wait at a traffic light, and nearly any place you remember to do them. They can also be done while you are actually urinating. After you start to urinate, try to stop the flow. You may not be able to stop at first, but keep at it. You will know you are accomplishing your goal when you can stop before you are finished and then start again.

In a few weeks you may notice a positive difference in your bladder control and a better toned vagina. However, these exercises will not overcome a significantly prolapsed bladder, which requires surgery.

COUNTING SHEEP

Added to all the bladder chatter and other indelicate problems we've mentioned is insomnia. Sleep disorder can happen at any age, but just when you no longer have to walk the floor with teething babies, scare away childhood nightmares, or wait up for tardy teenagers, you can't sleep when you have the chance.

Again, I'm going to point you to your doctor. After you've

tried natural means such as drinking warm milk at bedtime, cutting out caffeine, doing relaxation exercises, thinking pleasant thoughts, and avoiding naps during the day—go see your doctor.

Don't use over-the-counter sleeping pills. Remember that advertisers, with their glossy promises, want to sell you pills. They'll claim almost anything, including the harmlessness of their product.

If you have gone for a long time without sufficient sleep, a good doctor will want to help you. He knows that prolonged sleeplessness can bring on psychological disorders as well as contribute to physical problems. He may prescribe non-addictive sleeping pills, and he may also put you on estrogen. Not every doctor is convinced that estrogen replacement alters sleep patterns, but many think so, and my own personal experience persuades me that it does.

CUCKOO OR WHAT?

The women in my survey indicated that, in spite of their difficult physical symptoms, psychological changes were often the worst.

A few years ago Dorothy told me that she was afraid to drive her car. A very capable woman, she had driven without panic in Los Angeles traffic for years prior to menopause. But now she was immobilized by fear—terrified to drive anywhere, even nearby for groceries or to the hairdresser.

Originally, Dorothy's work was within walking distance of her home. One year, however, to keep her position, she had to transfer to another location a few miles away. Her husband wasn't free to drive her, public transportation didn't go that way, and she knew she couldn't impose on friends. She was forced to tackle her problem.

Dorothy belongs to a church that believes God can move mountains, so she asked her caring friends there to pray for her fear of driving. She enlisted other friends to pray. (I was one of them.) She saw a counselor. She also saw her medical doctor. She began forcing herself to drive short distances. Today she is back to driving without fear. She doesn't discount prayer and counseling, but she also knows that her recovery coincided with being put on estrogen replacement.

I went through a period of a year or more when it was almost impossible for me to go shopping by myself. (This is a confession from a formerly enthusiastic shopper! And I usually had gone unaccompanied.) Instead of gladly going for the weekly grocery supply, I would wait days until Jim could go with me at the end of our work day. If I had to go without Jim, I could barely force myself to go out alone. When I did, I would quickly grab up only the most urgent necessities and hurry home again.

Most often, Jim would give up his relaxation time to help me get groceries. He was less eager to go with me for clothes, gifts, and the other items essential to family life, so I would put off those kinds of shopping as long as possible.

I'm now over that little bout of resistance to shopping alone. Having gone through it, I can better understand other women when they talk about the strange, new feelings and attitudes that have come over them since menopause. It may be that the lack of estrogen doesn't directly cause those situations, but they are part of the mix of stresses with which women at this phase of life are dealing.

At the same time as we find ourselves contending with unfamiliar emotions, shifting family and career roles, and adjustments in many other relationships, our bodies are undergoing drastic changes. The good, old days are not coming back; neither are the good, young bodies. But God has given us assets that the young don't have. Let's do what we can to develop those assets and to keep our bodies and minds as vigorous as they can be.

6
The Estrogen Question

Bev was a basket case. She was postmenopausal and most of her world was in disorder. She was still having horrendous hot flashes. She was jittery and flighty. When she wasn't crying, she was angry. She ached all over and wasn't sleeping well. She felt that younger people—especially her children— were, as she put it, "leaving me out, passing me by, treating me like an old shoe." She and her husband had seldom had sex in the last three years; when they did, "it hurt too much."

When Bev was younger, she was a happy, self-confident woman with good leadership abilities. She taught a neighborhood Bible study in her home and did all the nice, motherly things with her children in their school and community.

After Bev told me how bad life was now, I asked her if she

was taking estrogen. ("Taking estrogen" is the shorthand way of saying "receiving hormone replacement therapy," also known as HRT or ERT.)

"Oh, no!" she said, "You know that estrogen causes cancer."

MISINFORMATION

Unfortunately, Bev's information was inaccurate. But she was living by it. She was determined to suffer through all her menopausal mess—even if it meant a lot of disruption in her relationships—rather than risk cancer.

Bev is not alone. Thousands of women, and, sadly, some outdated doctors, are going by old information. It's true that in the 1970s, researchers discovered that women who used estrogen had a higher incidence of cancer. However—and this is very important—subsequent research has shown that estrogen, given in the *right dosage* and with its corresponding hormone, progesterone, is not likely to cause cancer. In fact, many studies proved that estrogen taken with progesterone actually *reduced* the occurrences of cancer.[1]

One such test is reported by Dr. Lila Nachtigall:

Our own study at New York's Goldwater Memorial Hospital of 168 women, half on estrogen/progesterone and the other half on placebos, indicated that ERT is *more* than neutral—it is actually protective.

Although the expected rate over a decade in this age group would be four or possibly five cases, there were *no* cases of breast cancer among the estrogen users while there were four cases among the control group who took the placebos.[2]

Dr. Nachtigall also reports that this same group of estrogen/progesterone users had no cases of endometrial cancer during the 10 years of the research, but the control group had one.[3]

I have studied research from scores of doctors and scientific investigators about the use of estrogen for menopausal and postmenopausal women. I also have reviewed medical journals and technical reports with the latest findings, talked with many gynecologists and family physicians, and attended that eight-hour medical seminar on the subject. I did this for my own information—and before I would say anything to you. I'm convinced that, except for a few women, estrogen is safe.

I do, however, want to go on record as saying that I am *not* pushing estrogen replacement for every woman. Some women are at risk. And estrogen isn't a quick fix for every physical or emotional problem. I do think, though, that many women and some doctors dismiss hormone replacement therapy without enough thought or correct information.

When we realize that estrogen helps prevent the dreadful results of osteoporosis and heart disease—which can only fully be recognized after it's too late—plus the agonies from atrophying vaginal and urinary areas, and the havoc produced by fluctuating emotions, we should thoughtfully consider its use. Instead of simply "toughing it out" and "trying to have enough faith to get through it," let's evaluate the advantages and disadvantages of hormone therapy.

POWERFUL INFLUENCE

More than most of us ever know, estrogen is a potent hormone in our body. It circulates in the bloodstream and bathes all our tissues. At puberty it influences the development of our breasts, genitals, fat deposits, and other sex characteristics. As we saw in Chapter 4, estrogen controls our menstrual cycles. Throughout the years of menstruation, it also influences our blood chemistry, vascular system, and bones. Therefore, when it begins to diminish during menopause, there are serious consequences.[4]

Prior to menopause, women are far less apt to have a heart attack than are men. After menopause, the incidence of heart attacks and other cardiovascular diseases in women climbs to equal that of men. Cardiovascular disease (CVD) is the leading cause of death in women after menopause. But there is hope! Strong evidence now shows that estrogen replacement protects against heart attacks and stroke.[5] Chapter 10 will discuss this more fully.

And then there's osteoporosis, the unbelievably painful bone disease that cripples one-third of American women over age 60. Did you know that at least one out of three women sustains a hip fracture before age 80? One out of five women over 60 who fracture a hip will die of complications.[6] Other bone fractures, including the dowager's hump, cause extreme pain for many other women. Chapter 9 will deal with osteoporosis in more detail, but we want to note here that estrogen replacement has been proven to prevent or lessen osteoporosis.

ERT ENDORSEMENTS

Many of the books authored by medical doctors in the '80s and after strongly recommend the use of hormone replacement therapy. If you are reading something that absolutely advises against it, check the date it was written. It was probably copyrighted in the 1970s or early 1980s. Some authors writing during that cancer scare were very fanatical and, of course, were writing on the basis of the information they had at the time. Unfortunately, some people are still making decisions based on that out-of-date information.

Of the books and journals I studied for in-depth details about estrogen, I would highly recommend *Estrogen: The Facts Can Change Your Life* by Dr. Lila Nachtigall and Joan Rattner Heilman. I choose this book because of the writers' qualifications and because the average woman can easily understand it without a medical education.[7] Other good materials are also listed in the *Bibliography*.

Some quotations for your notebook:

ERT is safe when used correctly in the new medically approved way. . . . Women who take estrogen tend to live significantly longer than those who don't.[8]

Proper hormone replacement therapy will be the norm of the future; now it can be given correctly. Furthermore, such therapy will save lives as well as vastly improve the lives of women who avail themselves of it.[9]

Estrogen has been indicted, put on trial and now vindicated. Or we might say it has been paroled into the custody of progesterone. The two hormones should be prescribed together in a cyclic fashion. . . . With . . . a few

... rare exceptions, every woman should take estrogen and progesterone after menopause to protect against osteoporosis and cardiovascular disease.[10]

In the very technical documents from the proceedings of the 1989 Symposium on Long-Term Effects of Estrogen Deprivation, these conclusions were reported:

It appears clear that estrogen replacement helps to prevent osteoporosis. . . . Recent data strongly suggest a cardioprotective effect of estrogen. This beneficial effect may become an additional indication of estrogen replacement therapy (ERT). Indeed, if current calculations are correct, the eventual number of lives saved as a result of estrogen might make protection against cardiovascular disease the major indication for ERT. . . . It was the consensus of the participants at this conference that overall ERT is extremely beneficial.[11]

A new medical publication to provide advice to gynecologists who care for menopausal women was launched in 1988. Each quarterly issue is filled with scientifically based articles by renowned and respected specialists. One editorial had this to say:

Market research tells us that only about 15% of all postmenopausal women receive estrogen replacement therapy. And, while the number of women entering the menopause has increased, this percentage has remained relatively constant over the past 20 years. Recognizing that estrogen deficiency occurs in 100% of all postmenopausal women, and not suggesting that all women after menopause require replacement, the question nonetheless is—what happens to the remaining 85%? . . .

We now know that menopausal symptoms must not be ignored. Even "asymptomatic menopause" may initiate silent, progressive, and ultimately lethal sequelae. Simply stated—you can't "tough out" cardiovascular disease and osteoporosis. Osteoporosis does not develop only very late in life or just before death—it starts with the onset of hot flushes.[12]

BUT BEWARE

Even though much support is present for ERT, some dangers still exist. Women who presently have, or who have recovered from, estrogen-dependent cancer generally should not take estrogen. Women with severe diabetes or certain liver diseases also may not be candidates for estrogen replacement. Occasionally, however, when such women's lives are also at risk from other problems caused by estrogen deficiency, a doctor may decide to administer—and carefully monitor—some forms of ERT. If you are such a woman, you certainly would want every one of your doctors working closely together on the situation.

Women without these diseases need to be alert and informed, but with an annual physical to check for cancer, you can feel safe in using ERT. If you have your uterus and/or ovaries, be sure to have your doctor perform tests to detect cancer in those areas, as well as your cervix and breasts. You also need to faithfully examine your own breasts for lumps every month.

Estrogen does not cause cancer, but it can accelerate the growth of cancer already present. Early detection is the key to a good prognosis for all cancer, whether or not ERT is being used. So, again, I urge you to have a doctor's examination at least once a year.

Actually, we have more to fear from osteoporosis and cardiovascular disease (CVD) than we do from cancer. Deaths caused by osteoporosis and CVD greatly outweigh cancer deaths for women our age. Besides the women who die, untold thousands suffer for years from other consequences of bone and heart disease.

My mother has been in dire pain for more than 10 years, and now is very disabled, due to osteoporosis. Because of her history and other risk factors listed in Chapter 9, I know that I am in great danger of the disease. One of the crucial reasons I have elected to receive ERT is to prevent osteoporosis.

Cancer is also much less a possibility if you are taking *progesterone* with your estrogen. This is an absolute must if you still have your uterus, and many doctors recommend it for women without a uterus for the control of fibrocystic breast disease. (Also, for your information, most doctors now suggest that you eliminate caffeine in your diet and take 800 IU—international units—of vitamin E daily to reduce fibrocystic symptoms.)

Estrogen *dosage* is also a factor in reducing the cancer risk. The recommended daily dose used to be much higher than it is now. By the way, birth control pills have as much as 10 times more estrogen than is given to menopausal women on ERT.[13] The new lowered dosages make estrogen replacement therapy much safer.

MORE WARNINGS

Some other health conditions occasionally are made worse by estrogen, but safe ways around most of these problems are now possible.

High Blood Pressure

Only about five percent of women experience a rise in blood pressure from estrogen taken by the mouth. Since kidney enzyme levels are responsible for hypertension, estrogen from a skin patch or vaginal cream (which bypasses the kidneys) does not contribute to high blood pressure. Therefore, a woman prone to hypertension no longer has to avoid ERT, putting up with hot flashes and other menopausal discomforts. Nor does she need to risk osteoporosis and heart disease.

Diabetes

Estrogen in low dosages usually does not affect diabetes; although you and your doctor need to carefully watch your blood-sugar tests. High dosages would be a problem for sugar metabolism.

Fibroid Tumors

Many endocrinologists and other specialists tell us that the new, low dosages of estrogen do not usually cause fibroid tumors in your uterus.[14] Although they can cause pain and bleeding, small ones will shrink as estrogen declines with menopause. If they are very large and painful, you may need a hysterectomy.

Gallstones

Previously, women with gallbladder disease could not use ERT for relief from menopausal symptoms because estrogen tends to thicken and concentrate the bile produced by the liver. Now that estrogen can be received by way of a skin patch or vaginal cream, the liver is bypassed and estrogen will not cause the formation of gallstones.[15]

Liver Dysfunction

A damaged liver from some types of disease may not properly metabolize the estrogen that passes through it, so a woman with liver impairment should not take oral estrogen. But, again, help for her menopausal problems is available by using a skin patch or vaginal cream that transmits estrogen directly into the system without using the liver.[16]

Blood Clotting

Women who have a history of blood clotting (thrombophlebitis or thromboemboli) should be very carefully evaluated for the use of ERT. If estrogen is badly needed for other symptoms, a doctor may administer a very low dose of estrogen and then test the blood to see if it has affected the blood clotting factors. Since clots in blood vessels are life-threatening, estrogen may need to be avoided by these women.[17]

THE GOOD NEWS

After discussing the possible problems of estrogen replacement therapy because of some medical conditions, we may need to be reminded of why we wanted to take it in the first place. Of course, we have mentioned these throughout the book, but let's briefly review some of the advantages of ERT here.

Hot Flashes

The vasomotor system becomes unstable with the decline of estrogen, and one of the first, most noticeable symptoms is hot flashes—also known as hot flushes or night sweats. A few women are not bothered by hot flashes and decide to ride them out. Most women, however, find them very uncomfortable, disruptive to work and sleep, and embarrassing in public. Sometimes a hot flash also drains your energy, leaving you exhausted.

Hot flashes seem to be one tangible symptom that will help a doctor pay attention to what you're saying about menopausal troubles. I vividly remember one time when I unknowingly used the "magic words."

I had spent three or four visits with a doctor, asking about my painful periods, my creepy, crawly skin, my new aches and pains, and my emotional ups and downs. He gave a pelvic exam, did a Pap test, and checked my breasts, but he didn't seem to hear my complaints.

I had hot flashes, but they were less bothersome to me than my other problems, so I had forgotten to mention them on the earlier visits. That day I again was not getting much help, and then I just happened to say, "I've also been having hot flashes." Immediately the lights flashed and bells rang! (Figuratively, of course.) The doctor grabbed his prescription pad and told me I needed estrogen.

Other Vasomotor Symptoms

Estrogen replacement also helps stabilize the other vasomotor problems, which include heart palpitations, nervousness and irritability, strange skin sensations, and perhaps even insomnia and dizziness. These symptoms can have other causes, as you know, so you need to have a caring doctor help you be sure of the sources and the right treatment.

Skin, Membranes, Tissues, and Hair

Many doctors and researchers are enthusiastic about the positive effect of ERT on skin and tissues. Natural aging, sun, nicotine, and other factors all take their toll, of course, but the health of a woman's skin, membranes, and tissues are strongly related to her estrogen level.

Dr. Lila Nachtigall reports a 1985 British study that showed skin condition depends more on the age at which menopause occurred (and estrogen declined) than on chronological age. Another study found that the skin of women nearing 60 who do not take estrogen is only half as thick as those who do.[18] Estrogen nourishes the layer of fat just under the outer surface of the skin, which provides the skin with "inner support, firmness, and resilience." Estrogen also maintains water in the tissues and helps produce oil for lubrication. In addition, it keeps collagen, the connective tissue of the skin thick and firm. Without it, the skin wrinkles more easily.[19]

The inner membranes, such as in the vagina, also need estrogen for lubrication and padding. Even if you don't care if your hands and face are drying up, you may need ERT in order to to avoid vaginal burning and irritation and to have a good sexual relationship with your husband.

Estrogen controls the pattern of your hair growth, encouraging it on your head, pubic area, and underarms, and discouraging it elsewhere. After the loss of estrogen at menopause, your hair may get thinner, straighter, and drier. You also may start to grow hair in places you don't want it, such as on your face.

Vaginal and Urinary Areas

In addition to poor vaginal secretion, the decrease of estrogen causes the lining of the vagina to become thin and less elastic. The vagina eventually becomes short and narrow, returning to the size and shape it was before puberty. The dryness and thinness of the vaginal walls may result in inflammation, bleeding, and more frequent infections. With thin walls, no lubrication, and a small vagina, intercourse becomes painful and perhaps impossible.

Loss of estrogen causes the portion of the urethra located above the vaginal opening to thin and become more rigid. It is more easily irritated and infected. The distance between the vagina and urethra decreases, so that infections are more readily exchanged between the two areas.

These problems alone are enough to make you want to take estrogen! Anyone who has ever suffered through a urinary or vaginal infection never wants one again. Yet, many women endure one infection after another.

Aches and Pains

Osteoarthritis is the name given to those pains you may be feeling in your joints, although the problem is not actually arthritis, or inflammation of the joints, as the label suggests. It is a degenerative joint or bone disease that occurs twice as often in women as in men.

You *have* noticed lately that your joints hurt more, haven't you? You also may have much more muscle and back pain because of estrogen deprivation. Estrogen helps maintain muscular strength, bone density, and the protein matrix of your spine. If your estrogen is deficient, you're in for more pain.

Many researchers recognize the relief from joint and muscle pain that ERT gives, although they are not yet sure of the connection. Says Dr. Nachtigall, "We do know, however, that after about two weeks of treatment, ERT often dramatically relieves both muscle and joint pains."[20]

Cholesterol

Estrogen has another benefit. It raises the levels of high density lipoproteins (HDLs), which help lower the occurrence of clogged arteries and coronary heart disease. It also lowers the low density lipoproteins (LDLs), which are associated with the higher incidence of coronary artery problems. So estrogen therapy helps control your cholesterol and lower your risk of heart problems.

There's a catch, however. Progesterone can have the opposite effect by lowering HDLs and raising LDLs. So if you are on hormone replacement therapy that includes both estrogen and progesterone, it is important to have your cholesterol checked regularly and to have your doctor work with you on the right balance of estrogen and progesterone.[21]

Alzheimer's Disease?

More research needs to be done, but some early reports indicate a link between estrogen deprivation and Alzheimer's disease. Dr. Howard M. Fillit in an address entitled, "Hormones and the Brain: The Neuroendocrinology of Aging, Alzheimer's, Stress, Depressive Illness, and Appetite Disorders," gave encouraging news that perhaps estrogen replacement will deter Alzheimer's disease and other memory loss.[22] I personally would be glad if it does since some of my family members have been Alzheimer's victims.

Dr. Philip Sarrel and Lorna Sarrel also report that hormone therapy helps with short-term memory lapses. Women who misplace things, forget why they called someone, or lose their train of thought in a conversation improve with hormone therapy.[23] Around our office, when we can't remember what we're supposed to do or where we put something, we jokingly call it "sand brain."

Osteoporosis and Cardiovascular Disease

Both of these diseases can endanger our future health. We can grin and bear hot flashes until they're over, we can use antibiotics and lubricating jelly to help with our vaginal and urinary problems, aspirin will relieve our aches and pains, but the consequences of osteoporosis, heart attacks, and strokes are often fatal and certainly debilitating.

At this time, little is known about how to reverse the conditions once they have developed. And we are assured that they relentlessly begin their onslaught as soon as our estrogen begins its departure. Some women are more at risk, of course, and we will discuss this in Chapters 9 and 10. ERT seems a little like an insurance policy against two very probable threats.

Life Expectancy

You can plan to live longer if you are taking estrogen after menopause. You will be less apt to be one of the 30,000 women who die each year because of complications from osteoporotic fractures.[24] Your risk of death from heart attack and stroke will be lower, and you can expect an increase in longevity because of better overall health from estrogen.

QUESTIONS, ANYONE?

We should talk a little about dull things like possible side effects from ERT. We need to be aware of—but not terrified by—them. They are generally insignificant and temporary.

A few women experience nausea when they first begin ERT. This usually passes, but if it does not, perhaps it will help to take your pill at bedtime. Or try the skin patch or the vaginal cream that eliminate estrogen passing through the stomach.

Your breasts may become tender at first, but this usually diminishes in two to three months' time. If not, you may want to consider a lower dosage.

Fluid retention is a problem for some women using ERT. Your system will probably stabilize in a short time. Cutting down on salt intake will help. Some doctors recommend diuretics, but be careful. Diuretics can throw off your blood chemistry and cause more problems, such as weakness.

Because of water retention, you may temporarily weigh more. Some researchers claim that estrogen makes no difference in true weight gain; others say it does. The answer isn't final. But, remember, our metabolism is naturally slowing down, contributing to weight gain, and our body shape is changing. Estrogen actually helps us keep our feminine figure by controlling the places where fat is and is not distributed.

Some women experience a vaginal discharge because the hormones stimulate an overabundance of lubrication. Although a nuisance, this is not a medical threat.

Headaches may bother some women when they first begin ERT. If they are extreme or persist, you will want to get help, including the possibility of changing your dosage or form of estrogen.

Some women on ERT occasionally find that areas of their skin have picked up a strange pigmentation. Moles may get darker and larger, or tiny, benign tumors may appear in some places. Again, these may be undesirable, but they aren't dangerous. I have discolored patches on my neck by my jaws just below my ears. They look like a blotchy suntan, but I'd rather have them than osteoporosis.

A few women have an allergic reaction to estrogen, which is manifested by rashes, swollen tongue, and itching. Switching to another brand of hormones or trying another type of ERT (skin patch rather than pills, or injections rather than vaginal cream) may alleviate the allergy.

If estrogen and progesterone are being taken by a woman who still has her uterus, she may have monthly withdrawal bleeding for a time. This is normal, and even while on HRT, this should eventually stop after a few years. If it doesn't, or if bleeding occurs at irregular times during the cycle of the hormones, you must let your doctor know.

Don't let the regular bleeding discourage you from taking hormones. I know you want to be finished with all that, but the benefit of estrogen for your health outweighs the scant bleeding. If your bleeding is heavy or painful, you must see your doctor.

HOW MUCH ESTROGEN?

Your doctor, of course, will guide your estrogen dosage, but it helps if you are informed. The recommendation from most medical practitioners is the lowest dosage possible that will effectively care for your needs.

Postmenopausal endocrinology is still an inexact science, and since every woman has a different sensitivity to estrogen, be prepared to work at determining the right amount. If one dosage doesn't take care of your symptoms, be sure to let your doctor know. Some women complain to others that ERT isn't working when they need, instead, to be talking to their doctor so the best balance of hormones can be found.

Dr. Lila Nachtigall and others report that we need at least 0.625 mg of conjugated estrogen (conjugated estrogen is a combination of all three estrogenic hormones—estrone, estriol, and estradial) or an equivalent amount of other estrogen to prevent osteoporosis.[25] To care for hot flashes and other symptoms, the dosage may be increased if necessary.

The dosage of progesterone needed can be as much as 5 or 10 mg for seven or 10 days a month. My doctor and I have found that I can tolerate only 1.25 mg a day. Otherwise, approximately eight hours later, I have about an hour of very scrambled emotions. Not many women are affected this way, but, *again*, I say, "Work with your doctor."

WHAT METHOD?

Types of HRT include pills taken orally, injections, skin patches (transdermal patches), and vaginal creams. Perhaps by the time you read this, pellets inserted under the skin (implanted subcutaneous estrogen pellets) will be popular. Another method still under development is the vaginal ring implant. Researchers are continuing to look for the most effective method to receive estrogen, so it will pay for you to keep up-to-date. Your pharmacist, as well as your doctor, can tell you what is being most prescribed.

The skin patches are proving to be very successful for estrogen replacement. They are convenient to use and deliver estrogen at a controlled rate. A little patch similar to

a round Band-Aid is applied somewhere on the skin under
the clothing twice a week. A few women are allergic to the
adhesive on the patches, but that will probably be remedied
soon with a different adhesive. Some women are finding that
wearing the patches on their back or buttocks causes less
irritation than on their abdomen.

Both the patches and vaginal cream have the advantage
of bypassing the liver and digestive system, so that women
with preexisting health problems are not unfavorably affected. Estrogen in this form also is less likely to cause
hyperplasia (buildup of the uterine lining).

The disadvantage of vaginal estrogen cream is the
difficulty in knowing how much estrogen is actually getting
into the system. Also, vaginal cream alone is never sufficient
for protection against osteoporosis or heart disease. However, cream is sometimes the only way some women can
receive ERT. It is frequently prescribed to be used temporarily and in conjunction with another method of ERT.

Intramuscular injections of estrogen are less often used
than formerly. They have the advantage of delivering estrogen quickly to the system, but the disadvantage of allowing
the estrogen level to drop in a few days. Some women still
receive estrogen in this way, if the other ways are ineffective.

With all the methods of receiving estrogen, progesterone
is still needed by mouth or injection. So, if you elect to use
the skin patch or vaginal cream, don't forget to take your
progesterone as prescribed.

HOW LONG?

Several of the doctors who are most in the know about
hormones and their effect on our health recommend that

estrogen replacement be taken for life.[26] Others say at least seven to 10 years.[27]

Until his retirement, I was seeing the same physician who had treated Dr. James Dobson's mother during her menopausal trauma, which Dr. Dobson describes in his book, *What Wives Wish Their Husbands Knew About Women*.[28] One day as the doctor was talking to me, I heard a little beep from a car horn in the parking lot. He interrupted his consultation with me to explain, "That's my wife honking good-bye. She was here to get her monthly estrogen shot. She's 65 now, and I plan to prescribe estrogen for her good health for the rest of her life."

· You and your doctor will need to determine how long to continue hormone replacement therapy. You need to be warned that if you decide to stop HRT at some time, you should never quit abruptly. Your system won't be prepared for the sudden change, and you may experience severe symptoms.

WELL, WHAT'S YOUR DECISION?

I hope you will carefully weigh all the advantages and special considerations of hormone replacement therapy for you. Consult with your doctor—more than one, if necessary. Talk to other menopausal and postmenopausal women. Read. The library has many books on the subject. Check the qualifications of your sources, including your doctors, the authors of what you read, and the people to whom you listen. Remember to keep your future health in mind also.

Don't forget to ask God for his wisdom about the mat-

ter.[29] After all, he created you and promised to guide you. He
has also given medical technology to be used for our benefit.
Today we have no reason to suffer menopausal symptoms.
"After all," my gynecologist told me, "you don't earn Brownie
points for putting up with needless pain and discomfort—
not from your family or friends or even from God."

7

Hysterectomy— Pro and Con

I have a friend I'll call Doris whose cure for many health problems is, "Get rid of it. Cut it out. Whack it off." If someone has breast lumps (even though they are not malignant), Doris says, "Simply remove the breast and then you won't have to worry about cancer."

If you have a tooth that needs expensive repair, Doris would tell you, "Get it pulled." When I was wrestling with painful fibroids in my uterus, Doris urged me, "Have a hysterectomy and end all the agony."

One time, after listening to another of her she-should-just-have-it-removed lectures, I said, "Doris, I've been having a terrible headache for days . . ." She must have caught herself, because she didn't follow up with her usual solution!

"GET RID OF THE THING!"

We should not just blithely have our uterus removed to avoid uterine cancer, fibroid tumors, or pregnancy. A hysterectomy is major surgery, with the accompanying risks and side effects. We need to get all the information we can before making a decision either way.

Some facts to consider:

- One-third of all American women have a hysterectomy by age 65. The average age is 43.[1]
- Unnecessary hysterectomies are performed on as many as 30 to 50 percent of the women, according to some statistics,[2] and at least on 15 percent, according to more conservative reports.[3]
- If we live in the South, we are 1.7 times more likely to have a hysterectomy than if we live in the North. If we live in the Northeast, we are the least likely of all. No, geographic regions don't cause the need, but the medical "trend" is greater in some locales.[4]
- Nonsurgical methods are effective in dealing with many of the problems for which a hysterectomy is often advised.[5]
- A hysterectomy is not a simple method of birth control. Some husbands look forward to their wife's hysterectomy, thinking she will now be "more available." Such men don't realize the drastic effects of the lack of estrogen on her body.

A LITTLE MORE BIOLOGY

We also need to know some simple definitions and facts about surgical procedures. Many of us don't understand what is removed during surgery and what the effects will be.

A *simple hysterectomy* means that only the uterus and cervix are removed. Because the ovaries remain, estrogen is still produced, if menopause has not occurred prior to surgery. Menopause will usually take place at the time it normally would, although sometimes the shock of surgery does cause the ovaries to stop estrogen production immediately. Without a uterus, monthly periods end, and the chance of pregnancy is gone forever.

What some people call a *total hysterectomy* actually is a hysterectomy (removal of uterus and cervix) plus an *oophorectomy* (removal of the ovaries). The fallopian tubes are also removed, so the procedure is called a *salpingo-oophorectomy*. A *bilateral* salpingo-oophorectomy means the removal of both ovaries and both sets of tubes. By the way, removal of both ovaries means instant menopause.

A hysterectomy can be performed either vaginally, or abdominally by means of an incision. The procedure depends upon the individual situation.

A *myomectomy* is an alternative to a hysterectomy for the removal of fibroid tumors. It is used if a woman still wants children; however, the tumors may recur.

If the need exists at the time of a hysterectomy, other procedures may be included. These may cover repair for a *cystocele* (a protrusion of the bladder into the vagina), *rectocele* (a protrusion of the rectum into the vagina), or a stretched vagina. An appendectomy may also be done at the same time. A patient is to be informed of each procedure to be performed and must sign her agreement for each procedure.

The form I signed before my hysterectomy at age 50 asked for my consent for "exploratory laparotomy, total abdominal hysterectomy, bilateral salpingo-oophorectomy, Marshall Marchetti-Krantz procedure." This meant that an abdominal incision would be made to remove my uterus, cervix, fallopian tubes, and ovaries. The Marshall Marchetti-Krantz procedure was for corrective bladder surgery at the same time.

It came as a little shock to me when I was asked to sign another form, acknowledging that the hysterectomy would "render me permanently sterile and incapable of having children." If I had been under 50 years old, my husband would have had to sign the form too. That regulation has changed now; only the patient is required to sign an "informed consent."

I WISH I'D KNOWN

I waited six or seven years from the first time a doctor suggested I have a hysterectomy. In the meantime, I had a D and C (*dilation and curettage*), which is done under general anesthesia. The cervix is dilated, the uterine lining scraped and removed, and the tissue examined under a microscope by a pathologist. I also saw at least six other doctors. (We moved to a new state, so I had to start over in my search for a helpful doctor.)

I continued to have heavy bleeding, debilitating pain, and periods for eight days every three weeks. I knew I had fibroid tumors that were increasing. I was using estrogen (without progesterone) for hot flashes and emotional fluctuations, but the tumors may have grown anyway without estrogen.

The last two doctors I saw convinced me that I certainly did need the estrogen and, since the tumors would probably keep growing, I should just have a hysterectomy to end all the problems. Besides, they reminded me, I no longer planned to have more children and my risk of uterine, ovarian, and cervical cancer would be gone.

I thought I was well-informed before I decided to go ahead with the surgery. Now I realize I had received most of my information from the doctors who suggested the surgery and from little leaflets found in their offices, which really only explained the procedure and not the aftereffects.

I knew what was to be removed and repaired, and I knew I would have to recover from the abdominal incision, which for me was from the navel straight down. I also knew that I should expect to take a month to six weeks to recover.

What I *didn't know* was that progesterone therapy might have relieved my pain and bleeding, even my mild hot flashes, without having surgery at all. My fibroid tumors may have simply dried up when I completed a natural menopause.

I *didn't know* the effects of estrogen being stopped suddenly. In fact, in spite of my search for knowledge, I knew very little about how crucial estrogen is to our body or that removal of the ovaries means such an abrupt decline in estrogen production.

I *didn't know* how drastic hot flashes could be. The ones I had experienced before were trivial. When I went for a follow-up exam shortly after I was released from the hospital, I was sure I had a fever. I don't perspire easily, but water had been running off me for hours. It turned out to be a huge, nonstop hot flash. I later learned that the doctor should have had me on estrogen immediately after surgery.

I *also didn't know* about the vaginal and urinary changes that would occur. In the following months my skin became unbearably parched. I wondered why my hair became thin, dry, and didn't hold a curl well. My fingernails became unhealthy and still are. (My toenails are fine; they must appropriate all the estrogen designated for nails!) My psychological state never had been so undependable.

These changes would have eventually happened with a natural menopause, but I didn't know they would move in so swiftly and unscrupulously following a hysterectomy. A natural menopause allows for the body to adjust gradually to the decline of estrogen.

RISKS OF SURGERY

According to Dr. Penny Wise Budoff, 30 percent of the women who have hysterectomies experience nonfatal complications, such as fever, wound infections, and bladder and bowel perforations that cause lifelong problems. Another 15 percent need blood transfusions, which cause a high risk of contracting hepatitis or AIDS.[6]

A Cornell University study revealed that in one particular year, approximately 1,700 deaths resulted from 787,000 hysterectomies (.2 percent). The researchers also determined that at least 22 percent of those hysterectomies were unnecessary.[7]

Although the doctors with whom I consulted agreed that complications do arise and that unnecessary hysterectomies are performed, they felt that these figures were too high. One suggested that the statistics today are more like less than 5 to 10 percent for unnecessary hysterectomies. The point is that there *are* risks with any surgery, and the results of ovary removal (and, thus, the loss of estrogen) are not to be taken lightly.

REASONS FOR SURGERY

But some hysterectomies are absolutely necessary! Dr. Herbert Keyser, author of Women Under the Knife, issues stern warnings about needless surgery but recognizes that at times a hysterectomy is appropriate. He lists six situations:

1. Cancer of the cervix, uterus, ovaries, or fallopian tubes.
2. Diseases of the tubes and ovaries where the uterus is not primarily involved but must be removed because of its closeness to the diseased areas.
3. Involvement of the uterus in non-gynecological diseases such as cancer of the colon or a severe infection (abscess) secondary to diverticulitis.
4. An obstetrical catastrophe such as uncontrollable bleeding after delivery, uterine rupture, or massive infection.
5. Severe prolapse of the uterus.
6. Some cases of fibroid tumors of the uterus.[8]

Dr. Keyser notes, "The decision to remove the uterus for the first four conditions listed above is usually clear-cut and noncontroversial—and involves virtually no abuse by doctors. The last two, however, are the objects of much abuse; great care must be used to determine whether surgery is needed."[9]

TELL ME, DOCTOR

If you are contemplating a hysterectomy, be sure to get more than one opinion. You should also get the opinion from at least two doctors who don't know each other. Doctors often make referrals to other doctors with the same philosophies.

Following are some questions to ask:
- Why is the surgery necessary?
- Is there any other effective nonsurgical procedure?
- What, exactly, is a hysterectomy?
- Which type of hysterectomy is best for me?
- Will it be an abdominal or vaginal surgery?
- What are the possible complications of the surgery?
- What will be the side effects of a hysterectomy?
- Can I receive estrogen replacement therapy?
- How much time will I need to recuperate?
- How much will the surgery cost?[10]

SKY-HIGH

Surgery is expensive. The prices continue to rise so dramatically that it is useless to print a figure. If you are facing an operation, I would suggest you do as we did before my hysterectomy. In addition to asking about the doctors' charges, we inquired about the fees of the anesthetist, radiologist, laboratory, and any other costs.

Our medical plan allows us to choose hospitals, so Jim called all of them in our vicinity. He learned that the price of patient rooms and the operating room varied greatly among hospitals. We visited the hospitals with which we weren't familiar. We asked doctors, who weren't going to be doing the surgery, for their recommendations. We then made a decision based on cost, recommendations, and the atmosphere we sensed when we visited the hospitals.

AFTER SURGERY

Be good to yourself. Stay in the hospital for the recommended time. Enlist family and friends to keep your postoperative time as stress-free as possible.

Ask your doctor what to expect. Get specifics about going up and down stairs, lifting, bathing, sexual intercourse, driving, and returning to work. Ask other women who have had hysterectomies about their experiences in the early days after surgery. Glean the practical ideas and minimize the horror stories.

When you get home, have a comfortable place to recuperate. I had bought a set of perky, new sheets for our bed, to be used when I came home. Jim had the bedroom ready, roses from our garden greeting me, and everything I would need at hand. It became my special area for the next several days.

Allow enough time to recover. Dozens of women will tell

you, "Now is the most important time to take it easy. If you rest now, it will pay off later." You may give mental assent to the idea, but you'll be tempted to disregard the warning when some time has gone by.

I'd like to add my voice: "Take it easy!" You are the one responsible for yourself. As soon as you start back into activities, you will find it hard to stop. If people see you at church, they think you are back to normal. If you take on one little duty, you will be expected to take up all of your past obligations. You're the one who must monitor how active you should be. Don't let someone make you feel guilty if you know you must decline to do something.

Any major surgery leaves us weak for a time. On top of that, giving up our estrogen adds to our frailty temporarily, unless we start estrogen replacement immediately. Do what is emotionally nourishing for you to recover. Take care of yourself physically. Get all the medical help you need— medicine, guidance, and support.

You should know that you won't have all the post-hysterectomy symptoms all at once, and you probably won't ever have all of them. But don't be fooled. For the first year after my hysterectomy, I thought I only had the usual surgery aftermath to contend with. Most of the post-estrogen problems didn't appear until later. Then they surprised me by their vengeance. And there are the unseen violators, like osteoporosis and cardiovascular disease, that begin their work as soon as estrogen starts to depart.

GRIEVING

Mixed with the elation over no more painful periods and unplanned babies is a kind of grief. That, too, may not hit you for several months.

It was while I was coauthoring a book with our daughter who lost her leg to cancer that I realized that I am also an amputee.[11] My uterus, ovaries, and tubes were cut out of me.

Most of the time I have been more than glad to be rid of them, but sometimes I need to mourn a little. Other women tell me they do too—including older women who certainly did not want more children. Something has been taken from us. Like the healing process in any other loss, we need to allow ourselves to feel sad for a time.

Young women or single women who want to bear children perhaps have the most grief. I share the following poem a friend wrote. She is an unmarried missionary who loves children.

FOR WHAT MIGHT HAVE BEEN

It would have been an ecstatic conception.
Then, to know the being under my heart.
Oh, the thrill at the first sense of movement...
Possibly there would have been discomfort.
Then the increasing ungainliness of size.
Finally the pains would have come.
(They say it is the pain most easily forgotten.)
Joy and warmth with the nuzzling at breast.
The gift of the life-sustaining flow.
There would have been wonder at that little person.

No ecstasy—empty womb, bare breast.
Lord, channel that love and longing
    which YOU built into me.
Still my grief, renew my joy.
    Fulfill me as your person.
                    —Written on the eve of my hysterectomy[12]

JOY

After the emotion of that poem, I almost hesitate to share the next one with you. It was given to me by our daughter, Brenda, before my hysterectomy. She wrote it as a psalm, which turned my attention to God and his wonderful gift of three daughters who love him.

"LET HER REJOICE WHO GAVE BIRTH TO YOU."

Oh rejoice and sing!
Lift up your heart and praise the Lord.
Sing for the blessing which He has given to you.
Rejoice in the fruit of your womb.
Praise the Lord for the seed of your
    body has been multiplied;
    your seed has honored the Lord.
Be glad and do not hold your mouth shut from
    praising God.
Be glad and do not hold your tears of joy away from
    His presence.
Let your heart remember and ponder the fullness
    of motherhood.
Then lift up and rejoice!

"Behold, children are a gift of the Lord;
the fruit of the womb is a reward."
Psalm 127:3 [NASB]

"I have no greater joy than this, to hear of
my children walking in the truth."
3 John 4 [NASB]

Love, Brenda
July 24, 1984
Prov. 23:25b [NASB]

I have this handwritten gift framed and on the wall in a grouping of pleasant pictures and other mementos by our bed.

8
The Joy—or Pain—
of Sex

Norma wanted me to know that, for her, sex after menopause was great. She had undergone a hysterectomy three years earlier and she was reassuring me before my surgery. "I tell you, Bob and I have never enjoyed sex so much as we do now. Since my operation, I am instantly available. We don't have to bother with contraceptives. And there's no time of the month when I have to tell him, 'I can't because I'm having my period.'"

Four years later Norma was lamenting that her sex life was down the tubes. Oh, she and Bob still loved each other, but they were seldom having intercourse. When they did, it was usually unsuccessful. Her vagina was so dry that Bob couldn't enter. She ended up bleeding and hurting.

Norma had quit estrogen replacement therapy two or

three years after her hysterectomy. Her hot flashes were over and her nervousness had tapered off, so she felt she no longer needed estrogen. She didn't realize that slowly, but surely, her vaginal area was deteriorating.

She has now gone back on ERT, and if she responds the way other women do, her sexual relationship with Bob will return to normal.

Dr. Lila Nachtigall, the estrogen specialist who knows, says in bold print in her book: *Virtually every woman will eventually have to give up sexual intercourse unless she starts taking estrogen.*[1]

BETTER THAN EVER

The setting couldn't be better for a great sex life during the postmenopausal years. With no more fear of pregnancy, many women find themselves more relaxed and desirous of sex than they ever were with contraceptives. Not even considering the bother birth control was, just the fear that their method might fail was enough to keep some women on edge. And that's not a very good place to make love!

And there was the inconvenience. They told themselves contraception was worth it, but it certainly did dampen the romantic mood to have to climb out of bed and put in a diaphragm, or have their husband put on a condom. If the diaphragm-wearers prepared ahead of time, they had an emotional letdown if intercourse didn't happen.

If they were using a natural birth control method, they had to figure out whether or not the time was safe. I.U.D.-

users, having heard the horror stories of unwanted pregnancies and bizarre health hazards, felt uncertain.

Women who used birth control pills found more freedom, but they did have to remember to take the pills regularly. By age 40 they were told to suspend their use because of an increased cancer risk. They then had to find another method.

By not having to worry about birth control after menopause, having sexual intercourse is much easier.

By the time menopause occurs, the children in most households are gone, or nearly so. This means more freedom: the couple can leave their bedroom door open, go to other places in the house, make all the sweet love sounds they want, and skip the nightgowns and pajamas.

By this age, both husband and wife know more about how to make sexual intercourse a joyous and satisfying time. They know that sometimes lovemaking is soft and calm, other times more vigorous and aggressive. One time the husband initiates, another time the wife does. Some weeks they have intercourse many times. Other weeks they may skip altogether.

They may have sex morning, noon, night, or in the middle of the night. They often just hold and massage each other without having intercourse. They now know more about what pleases the other, and—sex manuals aside—whatever they choose to do is normal for them.

Sounds like a fairy tale, you say! No marriage is that ideal, of course, but some are closer to it than they've ever been before.

SOUR NOTES IN THE LOVE SONG

Unfortunately, just when everything should be going so well in their sexual relationship, some couples' union may be getting tattered and torn. They may find the empty nest very scratchy. "Just the two of us alone together" might not be as sweet as it sounds in the song.

When there's finally physical freedom, there's sometimes emotional strangulation. A mid-life crisis may confuse the husband's perceptions. Menopausal symptoms may turn the wife into an old battle-ax. Baggage from the past may appear on their doorstep, or problems with career, adult kids, or aging parents may short-circuit intimacy. One or both of them may think love is gone.

If this happens, the couple needs help for both the emotional and spiritual parts of their relationship. They may require professional guidance from a marriage-restoration-minded counselor. They may need to commit themselves to reconstructing a marriage different from what it has become over the years. They will need to start working to understand what each other's needs are at this new stage of life.

In our years of working with married couples in trouble, Jim and I have found that it isn't wedding vows that keep two people together. Even common bonds with children, work interests, or a strong Christian commitment may not be enough to help them stand the strain. They stay together when they are meeting each other's needs.

If they are malnourished inside, they will go—maybe unconsciously—to where their needs will be met. That doesn't always mean one goes to a "third person." But it does mean they start pulling apart from each other, here and there, in little or big areas, until the tear is extensive.

But there's hope! Many, many couples have learned how to renew their marriage and make it better than ever. It takes work, but it's worth it. If your marriage needs help, you might like to read *Your Marriage Can Survive Mid-Life Crisis: Ten Keys to an Intimate Marriage*, which Jim and I wrote from our own experience, from counseling other couples, and from an extensive survey of 186 couples who shared what had held their marriage together over the years.[2]

Some tips for restoring a deteriorating marriage are these:

1. Don't consider your marriage hopeless, even if there has been serious conflict, an affair, separation, or divorce.
2. People change slowly, but they do change.
3. Bad patterns of living or mistrust can be unlearned.
4. Let your mate handle his or her past—don't act as parents to each other.
5. The sexual relationship will grow as you confidently begin the courting process again.
6. Give authentic expressions to your current expectations and desires.
7. Forgive and release the past.
8. Enlist outside help.[3]

OLDER AND BETTER

If the feelings between mates are going well, their sexual relationship after the wife's menopause will survive too.

Menopause brings inevitable physical changes that can affect sex, but when the emotional wheels are rolling smoothly, a couple can better handle problem places in their sexual life.

We've already explained the vaginal changes that come with menopause in previous chapters, but in case you came to this chapter first, a quick review is in order. We'll even throw in a new word for the faithful folks who started at the beginning: *dyspareunia*.

Dyspareunia means pain with intercourse. Now you have an official term for the tearing, bleeding, and actual agony you may be experiencing with intercourse. Most likely, you did not have this problem before menopause.

With the menopause comes the eventual deterioration of the vaginal area. The walls become thin and lubrication diminishes or disappears altogether. The skin around the vulva becomes thin and dry so that it is more sensitive to irritation. In time, the vagina returns to a little-girl state, becoming shorter and narrower.

No wonder intercourse becomes painful and impossible! Now we know why all those stories and innuendos circulate about postmenopausal women not being interested in sex.

I am reminded of Edna whose husband, Bert, has been ignoring her for many years. In public he makes a fool of himself flirting with other women. He can't flatter them enough, yet he says nothing complimentary to, or about, Edna. He is eager to hug other women, help them with their coats, or help them in and out of the car. Edna can fend for herself.

Sadly, to many of his friends Bert makes no bones about

the fact that he and Edna have not had sexual intercourse for years. He accuses her of being cold.

The truth is, Edna had a hysterectomy many years ago. She is proud that she "never had to take estrogen or anything." She admits she can't have sex now, but she figures that's just something she had to give up because of surgery.

Apparently, down through the decades, many women have had a similar attitude. They may regret that their physical ability to have intercourse is gone, but they've decided they can do nothing about it.

But, again, there's hope! Sexual intercourse *can* be better than ever after menopause; however, as Dr. Nachtigall and many other doctors say, estrogen is a must. Vaginal atrophy can be stopped and even reversed with ERT. Some women still produce enough estrogen in their fat tissues so that they do well without adding more. Most women, however, need to replace the estrogen their bodies no longer make.

Without estrogen, many women not only experience pain and bleeding during intercourse, they don't even desire sexual intimacy. Seventy-five percent of the women in my study reported that they had experienced a loss of sexual desire. Many of them said it definitely had caused a problem in their marriage. I would say that 75 percent of over 400 marriages without the wife's desire for sex is cause for alarm! No one is quite sure how the libido is affected by the lack of estrogen, but we do know that when it wanes and ERT is introduced, a marked improvement takes place for most women.

The deceptive part about estrogen deficiency is that it may take years to show itself. A woman may think she is getting by, and she might—for five, or 10, or even 15 years.[4] Whenever she finally discovers she needs help, though, it is never too late for estrogen. Estrogen replacement therapy can begin at any age, no matter how long ago the meno-pause occurred.[5]

PRACTICE MAKES PERFECT

Actually, we should say, "Practice *keeps* perfect." I'm sure you've also heard, "Use it or lose it." That turns out to be true about a woman's sexual abilities after menopause. In addition to estrogen replacement, the best way to enjoy an active sex life is to have one.

Sexual intercourse keeps the vagina flexible, elastic, and lubricated. Being stimulated in this way—at least once or twice a week, according to Masters and Johnson—keeps the secretions going, aids muscle tone, and helps retain the shape of the vagina.

Dr. Nachtigall says that sexually active women have "a few years' leeway, delaying the inevitable changes until later in their lives. But eventually even they will have the same vaginal dysfunctions other women have—unless they use estrogen." [6]

SOME LITTLE EXTRA HELPS

Some women on estrogen replacement find they need additional lubrication to make intercourse comfortable, especially if they have had dryness for a long time. Water-soluble lubricants and vaginal suppositories are helpful, and they may be discontinued after the estrogen takes better effect. Of course, women who are not on ERT will need some kind of lubrication after menopause.

We are warned not to use products that aren't meant for lubrication. The perfumes and alcohol in some cosmetic lotions and creams will irritate already tender tissues. Petroleum jelly or baby oil may block our own secretions, and provide a breeding ground for bacteria. Vitamin E oil is acceptable, because it doesn't dry or cake and sometimes also relieves itching and irritation.[7]

As we've said, a doctor may prescribe estrogen cream to be used vaginally. Some of this cream is absorbed into the body, so a woman needs to be sure her doctor knows if she is receiving estrogen in another form. She doesn't want an overdose.

The cream is often used for only a short time until oral or transdermal estrogen takes effect. Estrogen cream actually restores the tissues of the vagina, causing them to thicken and become supple again. New non-estrogenic products that rebuild the vaginal cells are also now available without a prescription.

Another help to promote satisfying sex is to keep doing Kegel exercises. These are described in Chapter 5. Besides relieving mild cases of incontinence and toning up the vagina, the exercises stimulate desire. Some people even suggest doing Kegel exercises during intercourse to help provide pleasure.

Something else for a woman to keep in mind about sexual intercourse as she gets older is that her arousal and response times may become slower. So may her husband's. That's all right. If she has enough estrogen circulating, she won't have to worry about a deficient libido or lack of orgasms. It's just that timing is different.

Her husband may take longer to be ready to ejaculate; this gives more time for her to be stimulated. Occasionally he may not be able to maintain an erection or to have an ejaculation. That's okay too. She can afford to be patient and simply enjoy the pleasure of closeness.

If her husband continues to have sexual dysfunction, he should see a doctor. Some medications, such as that used to control hypertension, can affect a man's sexual ability. Stress, fatigue, and alcohol do too.

SAGGING SELF-ESTEEM

Sexual intercourse after menopause is directly affected by the physical changes we've mentioned, but it may also be influenced by the wife's changed body appearance. Yes, men age too, but their aging is considered less repulsive than a woman's. (Don't hit me! Don't hit me! That's what all the other women think, not what you and I think.)

In any case, a wife's self-esteem seems to be very fragile when everything about her body is slipping and sliding and creasing. What should be big gets little and what should be little gets big. Breasts decrease, hips and waist increase. The folds of old skin hide her once-beautiful eyes, but you can still see where they are by the dark circles.

She may become very self-conscious, especially if she knows her husband has an eye for the young, firm beauties that jog by them in the park or flaunt their near-nudeness at the beach. How can she possibly compete? She can't—if the basis for their sexual relationship is only what a young body can offer. Nothing will turn off her libido faster than feeling she is fifth-rate in desirability.

TURN PAIN INTO JOY

As I'm writing this, I feel as if I'm your friend. So I'm going to talk to you the same as if it were just the two of us sitting in our family room or on our patio.

If you need help with the emotional and spiritual side of your marriage, please do something about it. Don't just drift apart or wage war. Don't think divorce is an answer. Find a counselor. Read some books. Try to meet your husband's needs. Let him know what yours are.

Repair or nurture the friendship side of your marriage so that your sexual relationship will improve, if it needs to. Tell your husband how to be gentle with you when making love. Some men don't know how tender the vagina is when the skin becomes thin and there is little lubrication. Let him know ways to prepare you emotionally, by the little gestures and remarks he makes hours in advance.

Talk to your doctor about whether you should use hormone replacement therapy to improve your vagina and, perhaps, your libido too. Use lubricating aids if you need them.

Be the initiator some of the time. Think of romantic ways to set the tone for lovemaking. And remember that what you and your husband both enjoy is acceptable.

If either of you has a persistent problem, don't be afraid to get help. Talk to your gynecologist. Have your husband get a physical checkup. If necessary, see a sex therapist. Read some healthy sex manuals. Some that I suggest are listed in the *Bibliography*.

Sex after menopause can be super! It may differ from when you were young, but it can be *much* better. Even if intercourse isn't always electrifying, it can be pleasant and cozy. You may understand as never before that you are indeed one flesh. Intercourse is one of the nicest ways to express your love for each other. And there's no age limit to the enjoyment!

9

Osteoporosis— The Silent Thief

Osteoporosis is a wicked bone condition that, to some degree, sneaks up on every aging person. Its specialty is robbing postmenopausal women. It comes without an announcement and never leaves. Its arrival is quiet, but its activity devastating.

A simple, but graphic description of osteoporosis has been given by the doctors who wrote *Menopause and the Years Ahead*:

Osteoporosis literally means your bones are too porous. Because they have lost some of their calcium, they fracture easily. To make good concrete, you must have sufficient cement in the mixture. Less than sufficient cement (such as too little calcium in your bones) will produce concrete that will crack. Likewise, bones that contain too little

141

calcium also crack easily ... when your bones lose calcium, they lose strength.[1]

However, these doctors also tell us good news:

"We believe osteoporosis is a preventable disease."[2]

WHO CAN ESCAPE?

At least one-third—and some studies show one-half or more—of the postmenopausal women in the United States have been attacked by osteoporosis. A 1989 estimate placed the number of affected women at 15 to 20 million.[3] This many women would fill more than two cities the size of greater Los Angeles or greater New York City!

Men suffer from osteoporosis, too, but not to the extent that women do. For several years after menopause women lose bone mass about six times faster than men. By age 65 their loss rate slows.[4] Before age 80, one-third of all women will break a hip; one-sixth of all men will. Twelve to 20 percent of these fractures are fatal.[5]

Hips aren't the only bones that break because of osteoporosis. The other common sites are the vertebrae, forearm above the wrist, pelvis, and ankle. At age 45, men and women have the same number of wrist fractures; after 45 the number of broken wrists in women begin to increase until their number is 10 times more than for men.[6]

One-third of the women over 65 will fracture vertebrae.[7]

With one-third of the women breaking hips and another one-third breaking their vertebrae, that doesn't leave many unbroken women. Probably the remainder will break an arm, ankle, or pelvis!

In fact, Dr. Nachtigall says that 93 percent of all women who don't take estrogen will fracture a hip, forearm, pelvis, or vertebrae by the age of 85. Only one-third of the men will.[8]

All these facts and figures show how vulnerable you and I are to osteoporosis and its ravages.

ONE WOMAN'S STORY

I know a woman who was born when the 20th century was still a toddler. She has lived eight-plus decades in the clean, fresh air of the Midwest. She was unusually active and athletic as a girl, won high-school track meets all over her region (she still has the medals and ribbons to prove it), and earned every award there was to earn as a Campfire Girl in the days when Campfire Girls actually went camping.

In high-school home economics classes, she learned about the Basic Seven Food Groups. (Today they have been reduced to the Basic Four, but the same foods are still included.) She was so excited to learn what balanced eating could do for the body, she made sure she followed the Basic Seven religiously. Later, she made sure her husband and children did too. For the last six-and-a-half decades, and probably before, this woman has eaten right.

In her young adult years she was spry and agile. She taught elementary school for several years and spent many decades as the wife of a farmer. She got much of "exercise" doing outdoor chores. She bore and devotedly nurtured two children. She and her husband later moved to a small city where he had a cabinet shop and she worked in a large library. She waited on patrons, carried books, walked aisles, and climbed stairs and ladders all day. And she drank her milk, took vitamin and mineral supplements, and ate the Basic Seven.

Her menopause occurred sometime in her early 50s. Twenty years later the news about osteoporosis was out around the nation. A big campaign was launched to urge women to get enough calcium to help fight off this destroyer. This woman made sure she, too, got the recommended daily amount of calcium, in addition to taking other minerals and vitamins, drinking milk, and eating the Basic Seven. (Yes, I know it was four by then, but to her it was the seven.)

Before the calcium rage, this woman had begun to have unbearable backaches. But still she walked those aisles, climbed those steps, and lifted those books. She also did her own housekeeping and helped her husband with the yard work.

Her hips, legs, and shoulders began to hurt too. Over the next 10 or 12 years, she saw various doctors, most of whom said, "Take aspirin. Get enough rest. And eat right."

After a while she noticed that her shoulders and back were becoming very rounded. Every few days new pains shot through her spine—or hips and other places. She was in agony. She didn't sleep well.

In her 70s she retired from the library. About the same time, she bought a hospital bed so that she could adjust it to fit her crooked back. Later, making the bed was too painful, so she abandoned it to spend her nights in a recliner.

Her family encouraged her to do less bending and lifting

as she did her housework, but changing 75-year-old patterns is hard. When she was 76, her 82-year-old husband finally retired from his work. He was frail and could hardly walk. She lovingly became his legs and back. New pains, along with the old, kept grinding through her back, hips, and shoulders.

Specialists took X-rays of her spine that showed it to be terribly traumatized by little fractures. They pronounced her problem to be *osteoporosis*. They were sorry, but they could do little except to suggest large doses of aspirin or ibuprofen products.

By this time she had lost five inches in height. Her abdominal organs were getting crunched as she shortened and bent over. None of her clothes fit right. She was embarrassed to go shopping. She kept hoping that some day she could fit back into the "perfectly good clothes" in her closet.

Her husband died when she was approaching 78. She no longer had to care for him, but she missed him greatly. And her pain was with her constantly, even though she took massive amounts of aspirin. She would get out of her chair each morning, let her little dog out the back door, open the drapes, start breakfast, and need to sit again. She usually pushed herself beyond that, though, because she didn't want to "look like a baby."

She gradually could do less and less of her housework, but she wanted to keep her big lawn watered so it would look good with the rest of the neighborhood. She insisted on bending over to place sprinklers and drag hoses around the yard.

One morning at about 6:30 she hobbled to her backyard

in her housecoat to make some adjustments in the watering. After she bent down to screw one hose into another, she couldn't get up. She moved this way and that, but had no power in her back and hips to get upright.

She was determined not to stay there until someone came, which could be most of the day. So she crawled on her hands and knees, holding her housecoat out of the way. She managed to get across the back lawn, around one end of her house, and halfway across the front lawn to her front steps where she was able to pull herself up. The journey was painful—and embarrassing. By the time she got to the front yard, the biggest rush of early morning traffic was driving by her house!

This woman continued to live alone, becoming more and more disabled. She wanted to be independent as long as possible. Even though she spent much of her time in her recliner, with a heating pad, telephone, and TV remote control nearby, she still cared for her basic needs.

Some days, however, it was too difficult to get dressed. She shrank another inch or more; her digestive system became more dysfunctional in its tight quarters; and the bone and muscle pains were relentless.

By now she was beginning to hear that lack of estrogen caused osteoporosis. It was bittersweet news to learn that if she had received estrogen replacement therapy earlier, it may have prevented her situation. Estrogen would do nothing to restore her crumbled bones now.

Then the woman got shingles, a viral infection of the nerve endings, a disease as painful and distracting as osteoporosis. She was visiting her son and his wife at the time and is still with them because they've invited her to stay. The bout with shingles has passed, but the osteoporosis continues to eat away. She now spends hours in *their* recliner. And she still takes her calcium and vitamins, drinks milk, and eats the Basic Seven.

MY PERSONAL INTEREST

You've probably guessed by now that *the woman* is my dear mother. Her story illustrates only a little of the agony experienced by thousands of osteoporosis victims. Words on a page can never fully describe what they endure.

I hurt so deeply for my mother. I wish I could take her pain and handicaps and set her free. Even though the worst of the osteoporosis has been attacking her body for 10 years, I still am never prepared for the shock of feeling her shortened, bent, suffering body when I bend over to hug her.

At the same time that I hurt for her, I am concerned for myself. I want to do everything possible to avoid the same fate. According to the list of the factors most likely to result in osteoporosis, though, I am a prime candidate. My hope is to tip the balance of high-risk elements vs. preventive measures in favor of *my bones*.

NOT A BIT TOO SOON

Researchers are now making rapid advances in the study of osteoporosis. The puzzle pieces are falling into place as more is understood about the roles of estrogen, progesterone, parathyroid hormone, calcitonin, calcium, and vitamin D (and that's only part of the exciting list!) in the growth and repair of the body's bones.

These medical scientists are comprehending more about what makes bones deteriorate. They have determined that our genetic background, medical history, and daily habits play a part in whether or not we will fall prey to the disease. They are providing us with important prevention information and are coming closer to a breakthrough in reversing osteoporosis once it has set in.

Specialists have written entire books about osteoporosis. Yet I have room for only one chapter on the subject. So we'll look at only the most salient items of information so we can do our part to avoid or lessen the disease. Suggestions for further reading are in the *Bibliography*.

AT RISK

Following are some factors that help determine if you are likely to have osteoporosis. You will note that you can do nothing to control some of them—such as your nationality and complexion—but you *can* influence others.

If you have a score of 20 or more, you are in the high-risk category. Many doctors specializing in the prevention and management of osteoporosis would recommend that you immediately begin taking a daily minimum dosage of 0.625 mg of conjugated estrogen (or its equivalent) to stop the advancement of the disease.[10] As this chapter progresses, we will share other prevention techniques.

CHECKLIST OF RISK FACTORS FOR OSTEOPOROSIS[9]

	Risk Points	Your Points
Early menopause (before 40)	4	_____
Ovaries removed before menopause	4	_____
Family history of osteoporosis	4	_____
Northern European or Asian nationality	4	_____
Cigarette smoking (1/2 pack or more/day)	4	_____
Alcohol consumption (3 oz. or more/day)	4	_____
Small bones	4	_____
Very fair skin	4	_____
Diet low in calcium	4	_____
Eating disorder (anorexia nervosa, bulimia, etc.)	4	_____
Amenorrhea (no menstruation due to overexercise)	4	_____
Sedentary lifestyle	3	_____
Loss of height	3	_____
Recent fractures from minor injuries	3	_____
Underweight	3	_____
Hyperparathyroid disease	3	_____
Hyperthyroid disease	3	_____
Kidney disease	3	_____
Vitamin D deficiency	3	_____
Long-term use of cortisone	3	_____
Malabsorption problem	3	_____
High-protein intake more than 1 yr. as adult	2	_____
High caffeine intake (3 cup coffee or equiv./day)	2	_____
Adding salt to food at table	2	_____
Vegetarian diet	2	_____
Excessive high fiber diet (over 35-60g daily)	2	_____
Antacids with aluminum derivatives	2	_____
Bearing and breast-feeding at least 1 child	2	_____
TOTAL		_____

THEM BONES AIN'T JUST DRY BONES

Bones are not those quiet, lifeless body parts I always thought they were once I had reached my adult height. Instead, bone tissue is in a constant state of growth with new cells forming and other cells breaking down for reabsorption into the body. (Just so you can have some more big words to throw around, the "builders" are named *osteoblasts* and the "demolishers" are *osteoclasts*.)

Osteoporosis begins when the bones begin to lose more tissue than they make. The demolition goes on faster than the construction. Most people reach their peak bone mass before age 40. After that, everyone's bones begin to decrease a certain amount in density, strength, and toughness. Some people—women and men, adults and children—have health conditions earlier in life that allow osteoporosis to start, but the onset of the disease for the majority of people comes with the natural aging process or at the time of menopause.

Osteoporosis is currently divided into two types. One occurs in men and women at about age 70 to 75. It is thought to be caused by decreased production of vitamin D by the body, which is necessary for calcium absorption to maintain strong bones.

The other type of osteoporosis is most common in postmenopausal women. It appears to be caused by the decline of estrogen, which allows more rapid removal of bone. Also, after menopause, the intestines seem less able to absorb the calcium necessary for bone formation. So, less bone is formed while more is being removed.

YOUR "GIVENS"

You can understand that women who have smaller, less dense bones to begin with will be easier prey for osteoporosis. For some reason, women with fair skin are also more apt to get the disease. Therefore, black women and others with dark complexions are less at risk than women of northern European or Asian heritage. Black and Mediterranean women also tend to have much denser bones.

Women who have an early menopause or whose ovaries were surgically removed before menopause are also more likely to get the disease. Because they are without estrogen for more years, this allows the little demolishers to work longer while the little builders fall behind.

Family history of osteoporosis is also important. If your mother, grandmothers, or aunts have had serious cases of the disease, you are in direct line for the same—unless you take some massive defense measures.

Women who have suffered fractures from minor falls are suspected to be victims of the disease. If their height is beginning to diminish, they should also be wary.

MY "GIVENS"

I am half Danish, and the rest of my blood comes from Germany, Ireland, Scotland, and Wales. I was born a blonde with fair skin. My ovaries were removed at age 50. I don't know when a natural menopause would have occurred, but I may have had two to five more years of estrogen, skimpy as it might have been.

As I've told you, my mother has a serious case of

osteoporosis. Her mother and three sisters displayed moderate to strong signs of it too. My father's sisters have extreme conditions, with dowager's humps and fractures. One aunt fell and was hospitalized with a broken hip. Doctors determined that the bones had broken first, and then she fell. My family history is against me.

YOU'RE THE BOSS

Since you have no choice over your nationality, skin color, bone size, or time of natural menopause, what can you do? You can compensate by lowering the other risk factors as much as possible. Unless you are one of the few who shouldn't, you can use estrogen replacement therapy.

You can also take direct responsibility for many aspects of your lifestyle that affect osteoporosis:

- Don't smoke.
- Don't drink alcohol (or keep it to less than 3 oz. a day).
- Drink plenty of milk and eat dairy foods rich in calcium.
- Take calcium supplements so that your total daily intake is at least 1,500 mg (1000 mg if your ovaries are still functioning or you are taking estrogen).
- Eat a balanced diet with correct amounts of protein, carbohydrates, fats, fiber, etc. (Use a sensible nutrition book as a guide.)
- Get help to correct an eating disorder.
- Decrease salt intake.
- Cut down on caffeine to no more than the equivalent of 3 cups of coffee per day.

- Exercise, but don't overdo it.
- Ask your doctor if estrogen replacement therapy is a possibility.

You may have other health conditions or diseases that affect body functions or require medication that contribute to bone loss. But perhaps you can be involved in choosing the type and duration of treatment to lessen bone loss as much as possible. For example, if you must use cortisone or other steroids, let your doctor know your concern about osteoporosis. Maybe another remedy would be effective without causing bone deterioration.

WHY ALL THESE DO'S AND DON'TS?

Certain foods and substances that we take into our bodies either leach calcium from our bones, prevent the growth of new bone, or block the work of hormones, vitamins, and minerals to maintain healthy bones. A diet too high in red meat, for instance, causes too much calcium to be washed out of the body through the urine.

On the other hand, a strict vegetarian diet causes excessive loss of estrogen through the feces. Too much fiber in the diet "binds" calcium, preventing its use by the body. Salt and caffeine promote loss of calcium through the urine, while smoking lowers the estrogen level which, in turn, creates a high risk for osteoporosis.

Notice that some products increase destruction of existing bone while others reduce the formation of new bone. Alcohol is one that reduces bone formation, or the "osteo-blastic" activity. Dr. Kenneth Cooper says, "Every ounce of alcohol you drink has a negative impact on those cells that build up your bone structure."[11]

The December 1983 issue of the *American Journal of Medicine* noted that "alcohol consumption, along with cigarette smoking, was a major factor in promoting osteoporosis in the spines of 105 men ranging in age from 44 to 85 years."[12]

So the men you know who drink and smoke could be setting themselves up for a similar fate as a postmenopausal woman. (If one is your husband, please don't nag at him. Just suggest that he read the last chapter of this book.)

TWO MORE DO'S

Some other facts are important to know. *Exercise*, especially weight-bearing activity, is strategic to preventing osteoporosis. Walking, bike riding, running, jumping rope, or climbing stairs are good weight-bearing exercises. One or more of these should be done four or five times a week for about half an hour. Exercise, in some way not fully understood, stimulates bone cells to be more active and to produce stronger bone.

We must be careful not to overdo exercise, however, as has been learned from female athletes who exercise so strenuously that menstruation stops before menopause (amenorrhea). This means that the ovaries have stopped producing estrogen needed for healthy bones. Even after menopause we can exercise until we are too thin and put our bones at risk.

Heavier women have less tendency toward osteoporosis, probably because their bones are stimulated to grow in density to carry their weight. Also, their fat cells may be fostering the production of estrogen to help prevent bone loss.

In addition to the appropriate amount of weight-bearing exercise, *calcium* in our diet is a necessity. Since the need has been well-advertised by the calcium companies for years, we should be educated to its importance by now.

Following are some things to know about calcium intake:

- The suggested daily dosage is:
  1000 mg per day before menopause
  1000 mg per day after menopause with ERT
  1,500 mg per day after menopause without ERT
- It's nearly impossible to get the required minimum dosage entirely by drinking milk and eating dairy products. Pills or capsules are needed as a supplement.
- Calcium is best absorbed if it's taken throughout the day rather than at one time.
- Take extra calcium if you are on a high-fiber diet, since the fiber doesn't give the intestines time to absorb calcium well.
- Some leafy, green vegetables, such as broccoli, turnip greens, and collard greens are good sources of calcium. However, some other greens, such as spinach, beet greens, and Swiss chard, are actually *calcium blockers* because they contain oxalic acid. The calcium contained in those vegetables does you no good. And if you eat the blockers while taking in other calcium sources, such as milk, they actually prohibit the absorption of that calcium too.

YEAH, ESTROGEN!

As crucial as it is to receive sufficient calcium each day, researchers are discovering that calcium isn't enough. Exercise is important, as well as avoiding the no-no's, such as smoking and alcohol. But the single, most important deterrent to osteoporosis is *estrogen*. Once our body no longer makes enough of its own, replacement is needed.

Remember that my mother was very careful to eat well and was a very active woman. She never smoked nor drank a drop of alcohol. Probably her single biggest error was not having estrogen replacement after menopause. If she had only known about it!

A daily dosage of 0.625 mg of estrogen is enough to prevent osteoporosis before it begins, if the replacement is started immediately at menopause. If estrogen therapy is started later, it still will stop bone loss from progressing any further.[13]

That's wonderful news! I'm so grateful to the researchers for learning this in time for my generation.

BUT WHAT ABOUT SOMEONE ELSE?

However, some of us cannot take estrogen replacement therapy and others of us just don't want to use it, even if it *is* safe.

Some alternatives do exist. I suggest that you get more detailed help from such books as Dr. Kenneth Cooper's book, *Preventing Osteoporosis*,[14] Dr. Harris McIlwain's *Osteoporosis: Prevention, Management, Treatment*,[15] and other well-researched books from your library.

Just to whet your appetite, some of your options include another hormone known as calcitonin, the thiazide diuretic, sodium fluoride, and parathyroid hormone treatment. Of course, these aren't perfect either and can cause side effects. In the meantime, you also keep eating that balanced diet, getting sufficient exercise, and avoiding the stuff that's bad for you.

DETECTION

You may be thinking it would be great to know whether or not you already have osteoporosis. It's no comfort to realize that the surest way to know is after you've had a fracture.

Unfortunately, bone loss doesn't show up on conventional X-rays until about 35 percent has been lost. Other tests can be conducted to determine bone loss, but many researchers concede that none is yet completely satisfactory. Costs are high, results are inadequate, and availability is limited to medical facilities that can afford the equipment.

Photon-densitometry equipment and CT (or CAT) scanners may be the best for revealing osteoporosis at this time. If you are at high risk, you may want to have a baseline scan done now to judge changes in your bone density in later years.

Osteoporosis clinics are becoming more available around the nation, so if you live near one, you should be able to get some up-to-date guidance and care. Some hospitals offer community education programs. I would also suggest that you keep checking your library for the latest resources.

Because technology is changing so rapidly, rely only on current information.

Unfortunately, the best way to predict your likelihood of osteoporosis at the present time is based on the risk factors. As you go over the list, you will want to take active steps to control as many factors as possible.

The next time you watch a little, old lady with a dowager's hump slowly and painfully moving along somewhere, just decide that—as much as is in your power—you will not be the same in a few years!

10
Combating
Heart Attacks and
Other Assaults

Ellie was sitting in the evening church service with her oldest granddaughter. Suddenly she could no longer ignore the pains in her chest. She wasn't able to get her breath! If she could have, she would've screamed because of the sharp twisting pain in her heart.

All afternoon she had felt a strange tightness in her lungs or around her heart—she couldn't really locate it or describe it. She was also very, very tired, but she wanted to hear her pastor's evening message. Besides, she had promised to take eight-year-old Shana with her. Ellie wanted to encourage Shana's growing interest in spiritual matters, and she enjoyed having Shana beside her in church.

Ellie decided to go to the service and then rest as soon as she got home. Her husband stayed home with his elderly mother, who was visiting them for the weekend. She didn't mention her discomfort to John or his mother.

Ellie and Shana took seats near the front of the church. As soon as they sat down, Ellie realized that the tightness in her chest was strengthening its grip. "Oh, well," she thought, "I can stand it for another hour or so." She could hardly get up to sing the first congregational song, but she did. What a joy to be standing beside Shana who was singing with all her little being!

As the service progressed, Ellie found it very hard to concentrate. She was glad the congregation could remain seated after the first song. Then, just as a soloist got up to sing before the pastor would begin his message, Ellie's pains stabbed right through all her bravery.

Without any more arguing with herself, she got up from the pew and rushed out the door at the front of the sanctuary. She felt she was about to pass out and she wasn't going to do it in church. Shana sensed that something was terribly wrong, grabbed Grandma's purse and Bible, and followed her. A friend, noticing that Ellie was having trouble, also followed.

Shana and the friend helped Ellie to the church office, where she fell onto a couch. They tried telephoning John at home, but the line was busy. Next they dialed Ellie's doctor. No answer. Ellie was able to breathe a little better by then and didn't want everyone to get overly alarmed. But she finally agreed to let them call their small-town hospital. The nurse on duty advised the friend to bring Ellie right over.

In the hours and days that followed, tests revealed that Ellie had suffered a mild heart attack. She and her family were surprised. They thought only men and very old people had heart attacks. Ellie was just 50.

This couldn't be happening! She was a busy woman, with a flower and gift shop that was doing a booming business. It was two weeks before Christmas, and she had a lot to get done. Once she became stabilized and was over the extreme pain, she felt she had to get back to her work. Her doctors, however, insisted that she needed to rest and recover. Other people were enlisted to fill her place at the shop.

Ellie eventually had an angiogram, which showed that the blockage in her blood vessels was mild enough to be treated with medication rather than surgery. She was told to lose weight and lower her cholesterol level.

For over a year now, Ellie has had to modify her lifestyle. Although she still is overly committed many times, she is aware of that tight little warning that starts nagging in her chest, telling her she must cut back and rest.

DEADLY SITUATION

What many don't realize is that heart disease is the number one killer of women after menopause.[1] Heart attacks and strokes cause more deaths than either cancer or osteoporosis.[2]

Cardiovascular disease (CVD) is the term used for disorders of the heart and circulatory system. For nonmedical people like most of us, it is enough to know that CVD includes heart attacks, strokes, hypertension (high blood pressure), arteriosclerosis (thickening and hardening of the arteries), and atherosclerosis (a form of arteriosclerosis caused by excessive fatty deposits lining the arteries).

To understand the seriousness of the problem of cardio-vascular disease, it helps to see it this way:

For every 2,000 postmenopausal women, without estrogen replacement, in any given year,

- 20 will develop coronary disease and 12 will die from it;

- 11 will develop significant bone loss and one will die (probably from a hip fracture);

- six will develop breast cancer and two will die; and

- three will develop endometrial cancer.[3]

Therefore, although we should be concerned about osteoporosis and cancer, far fewer deaths result from these diseases than from heart and circulatory disease.

An alarming report has been issued by researchers for the American Heart Association following their study of the risk of heart disease for women over age 55. They find that by age 55, women are as likely as men to develop high blood pressure. By age 65, women are at greater risk for high blood pressure than men. A study of people ages 55 to 74 found that over half of the women have elevated cholesterol levels (which are a major cause for heart attack and stroke), while only one-third of the men do. Interestingly, a 55-year-old woman who smokes faces a greater risk of heart attack than a 55-year-old man who smokes.[4]

Time to stop and think! Most women have assumed that they were safe from heart problems, unless they were greatly overweight or had a family history of heart disease. It's true that few premenopausal women have heart attacks, but after menopause (when estrogen has impudently defected!), it takes only six to 10 years for women to catch up to men for heart attack risk.[5]

CAUSES OF CVD

The following factors increase the risk of cardiovascular disease:
- Aging
- Smoking
- Blood pressure
- Cholesterol level
- Glucose intolerance and diabetes
- Menopause
- Family history of CVD
- Excessive alcohol
- Oral contraceptives, *if you are over 35 and smoke*
- Obesity
- Physical inactivity
- Environmental stress[6]

How many of these are a problem for you? How many can you control? Wouldn't you like to stop the aging factor! Some items you can change; others you can't. If you drink or smoke, you should stop. You can exercise. You can watch your intake of saturated fats (most animal fats and some vegetable oils, such as coconut and palm oil).

You can even take responsibility to manage, or at least accept, the environmental stress in your life. (Environmental stress includes problems outside yourself that can cause inner stress: traffic congestions, noise, distance to shopping, weather, unapproachable boss—you have your own unique circumstances.)

While we mid-life women are concerned about all of the above conditions, in this book I am specifically interested in letting you know the correlation between menopause and cardiovascular disease. Every few months new findings are being announced about the powerful influence that declining estrogen has upon a woman's heart and blood vessels.

One of these reports was given by Dr. Leon Speroff at a conference on the effects of women's sex hormones on cardiovascular disease. He reported that "the ability of estrogen to lower serum cholesterol levels and, ultimately, the risk of cardiovascular disease, may prove to be a more important indication than osteoporosis for hormone replacement therapy in the postmenopausal woman."[7] ("Serum cholesterol" means the free cholesterol circulating in the blood.) Dr. Speroff is saying that it may be more important to prescribe estrogen replacement therapy to prevent cardiovascular disease than to prevent osteoporosis.

A research project known as the Leisure World Studies was conducted over a period of years with 8,841 women in a Southern California retirement community. The researchers found a 20 percent lower death rate among ERT (estrogen replacement therapy) users than among nonusers. The women using estrogen had 41 percent fewer heart attacks than nonusers.[8]

The National Institutes of Health published the results of research covering 2,269 women between the ages of 40 and 69 for a period of 5.6 years. The death rate among women who did not take estrogen after menopause was two-thirds higher than for women who did. Women who had their ovaries removed before menopause (causing a sudden halt to estrogen production) and who received ERT had a death rate 10 times lower than women who did not receive ERT.[9]

A LITTLE KNOWLEDGE IS BETTER THAN NONE

Since estrogen replacement lowers the cholesterol level, which in turn reduces the risk of cardiovascular disease, we need to learn some of the facts so we can intelligently care for our health. After all, it's *our* heart that may suffer the attack or *our* brain that may be left dysfunctional after a stroke!

Ellie is the one who lives daily with the aftereffects of *her* heart attack. While she is thankful it wasn't worse, she is limited in how much she can do and what she eats. Sometimes her business projects demand that she work long, pressure-filled hours. If she does, she pays for it with chest pains and the very real threat of another—perhaps more deadly—heart attack.

To better care for our cardiovascular health, therefore, we need to know more about cholesterol. Misunderstanding about it is rampant. Many of us don't actually know what "it" is, but we've been told it's bad. Of course, complete facts about cholesterol and its effects on our heart and blood vessels are very complicated. Since most of us don't have a medical education, I'll make the discussion easy to understand. While the information may be simple, the subject is *serious*!

Cholesterol Defined

Cholesterol is not simply *fat*, as many think. Cholesterol has a special chemical composition all its own. Fats, however, are contained *in* cholesterol. These fats (lipids) are *high density lipoproteins* (HDL), *low density lipoproteins* (LDL), and *triglycerides*. They are major risk factors for heart disease. More about these later. . . .

Cholesterol is not all bad. It's not a foreign substance; it is a basic part of our body. As is often the case for many of our body substances—the right amount of cholesterol with its components in correct balance is *very crucial* to our existence.

Cholesterol is needed for the health of our brain tissues, nerve sheaths, and other cells. It is vital for our hormones and body chemicals. It regulates the passage of substances through cell walls and acts as a conductor to transmit nerve impulses through the body. Cholesterol keeps us from becoming waterlogged when we are wet and prevents us from disappearing into thin air by evaporation.

Cholesterol is so important to our body that the liver manufactures it whether or not we get it in our diet. In fact, 70 to 80 percent of the cholesterol in our body is naturally present, no matter what we eat.[10] So, although we should guard against too much cholesterol clogging our arteries, we need to know that it is absolutely essential for our health.[11]

Cholesterol Tests

Cholesterol testing has become very popular. As one doctor explained to me, "There is mass hysteria about cholesterol." This is because we lay people do not understand the issue well enough, and product-pushers have taken advantage of us.

We are told that too high a cholesterol level is dangerous for the health of our heart and blood vessels. Medical experts say, however, that this may or may not be the case. Media and advertisers have oversimplified what is meant by "cholesterol level."

A test that only reports a "total serum cholesterol" can cause many of us to get needlessly frightened or, in some cases, lull us into a sense of false security. Our test can show a high cholesterol level when we are not actually at risk, or it can show a low cholesterol level and we can be at great risk!

As an example, a physician told me of a man whose cholesterol test showed a very low level when, in fact, he had already suffered many cardiovascular problems due to clogged arteries. His blood vessels were so lined with cholesterol, there was little left to circulate in the blood and show up in a test!

Because the results of a simple cholesterol test merely show a broad, general picture, doctors consider it only an initial screening tool, which may need to be followed up by a more complete *blood lipid profile*. Remember, cholesterol is present throughout our body, but most of it can't be measured with a blood test, including the cholesterol that is overzealously lining our artery walls!

A Truer Cholesterol Picture

What is more important in getting an accurate assessment of our danger of heart disease is to know the levels of our triglycerides, low density lipoprotein (LDL), and high density lipoprotein (HDL). Especially helpful is to know the *ratio* of our high density lipoprotein to our total cholesterol. This is known as the HDL Ratio, with which any physician should be familiar.

To be able to discuss these matters with a doctor, some more definitions are in order. Triglycerides are the fats, such as corn oil or beef fat, circulating in our bloodstream. High density lipoproteins (HDL) are known as "good cholesterol" because they carry away the plaque formed by cholesterol and triglycerides on our artery walls. Low density lipoproteins (LDL) are harmful because they take fat out of the blood and store it on artery walls and in other tissues.

So, we want to keep our LDL count low and our HDL count high. That's easy enough to remember: low density lipoprotein (LDL) should be low and high density lipoprotein (HDL) should be high! Triglycerides should also be low because that gives less fat in the blood for any sneaky little LDLs to store away to clog our blood vessels.

What's Your Score?

According to Drs. Sharon and David Sneed in *Prime Time: A Complete Health Guide for Women 35 to 65*,[12] these are the current recommended guidelines for acceptable levels of cholesterol and blood lipids for men and women of all ages as set by the National Heart, Lung, and Blood Institute:

Levels for HDL, the *good cholesterol*, should be high. As I've already indicated, many experts believe the most accurate picture of heart disease risk is the HDL ratio, which is found by dividing the total cholesterol level by the HDL level:

Cholesterol Level   **Risk of Heart Disease**
Less than 200 mg/dl*   =   safe level for all adults
200 to 239 mg/dl   =   borderline
Above 240 mg/dl   =   high risk
(*mg/dl means milligrams per deciliter. A deciliter is one-tenth of a liter.)

If the cholesterol level is greater than 200 mg/dl, further testing should be done to include LDL, HDL, and triglycerides.

LDL Cholesterol   **Risk of Heart Disease**
Less than 130 mg/dl   =   safe for all adults
130 to 159 mg/dl   =   borderline
Above 160 mg/dl   =   high risk

$$\text{HDL Ratio} = \frac{\text{Total Cholesterol}}{\text{HDL Cholesterol}}$$

The HDL Ratio should be 4.5 or less; the ideal is 4.0 or lower.

The recommended level for triglycerides is 200 mg/dl or less, with the ideal being less than 150 mg/dl. Tests for cholesterol lipids and triglycerides should always be done after fasting for 12 hours, since the levels vary greatly with the type and amount of food just eaten.

I would suggest that you have cholesterol testing done each year when you go to your doctor for a pelvic and breast examination. If you have a high cholesterol level, specific treatment to reduce LDH cholesterol is available.

NOW FOR THE GOOD NEWS!

How wonderful to know that estrogen keeps our HDL high and our LDL low! For the postmenopausal woman who can be on estrogen replacement therapy, this is reason enough to be on a lifelong program.

Dr. Lila Nachtigall says, "Can estrogen keep you alive longer? There is growing evidence that it can by improving the cardiovascular system and protecting you against heart disease. *Women who take estrogen tend to live significantly longer than those who don't.*"[13]

Estrogen replacement needs to continue for as long as we live.[14] Some studies demonstrate that past use of estrogen does not protect after estrogen replacement is discontinued.[15] Other major research also shows that the longer estrogen is taken, the more cardiovascular risk is reduced. In addition, their findings indicate that the dosage probably needs to be higher than 1.25 mg for the best protection.[16]

As I mentioned earlier, many tests have already proved the effectiveness of estrogen in preventing cardiovascular disease, and new studies continue to be conducted. If you are reading material that doesn't acknowledge this, you need to check the date. The information is out-of-date or the author misinformed. If your doctor isn't aware of the latest research, you should find one who is.

When I asked Ellie if her doctors had mentioned that her

heart problems may be connected with menopause and a lack of estrogen, she replied, "No, they just told me that it happens to 'women my age.'"

Sometimes doctors don't get very specific with us because they think we won't understand. You, of course, probably don't have a medical education, but you can be familiar enough with the key ideas to ask the right questions. For more information on major research and resources, please see the *Notes*.[17]

A LITTLE BIT OF BAD NEWS

As a friend of mine says, "Nothing is ever easy!" Estrogen is great for preventing cardiovascular disease. But estrogen needs to be accompanied by progesterone to prevent endometrial cancer and perhaps to control breast fibrocystic disease (see Chapter 6). Here's the hitch—progesterone is known to lower the HDL level and to raise the LDL level![18] In other words, some forms of progesterone (also identified as *progestin* in medical literature) negate, and may actually reverse, the positive effects of estrogen in protecting against heart disease.

But the news is not totally bad. Studies done thus far suggest that a *low dosage of progesterone* is enough to protect against cancer and not greatly affect the lipoprotein levels. Research is also being done to verify that some forms of progesterone do not cause a rise in lipoproteins. Early tests indicate that low dosages of newer progesterone formulations will not contradict the positive effects of estrogen.[19]

The answers are continuing to come in. For now, you can

ask your doctor to keep your progesterone dosage as low as possible and to prescribe one of the newer types of progesterone least likely to raise your lipoproteins.[20]

The evidence is so strong for estrogen protection against cardiovascular disease that I hesitate to even mention the progesterone caution. I don't want to scare you away from hormone replacement therapy. However, you are wise enough to be able to handle the complete information and to help your doctor make the best choices for your total health.

If you are a candidate for estrogen, *you should receive estrogen replacement along with a low dosage of progesterone.* You will then have a good defense against cardiovascular disease, as well as against osteoporosis and degeneration of your vaginal tissues. And, remember, there's also strong evidence that ERT improves your overall health.

SENSIBLE CHOICES

Of course, hormone replacement therapy doesn't substitute for a healthy lifestyle of correct eating, exercise, and eliminating smoking and drinking. Just imagine a cartoon of an overly obese woman in a cushy lounge chair in front of TV all day and night, week in and week out. When she isn't stuffing her face with food, she has a beer or a cigarette, or all three. But she faithfully takes her estrogen and progesterone and thinks she won't have a heart attack!

Many of us may not spend hours in a lounge chair, but we still put the wrong kinds and amounts of food and drink into our bodies while we rush around with our busy schedules. We are more active than the cartoon woman, but we have more stress. Our risk of cardiovascular disease may be as great as that of the inactive slouch. While we take our hormone replacement, let's realize it will do us more good if we accompany it with sane living—good diet, exercise, and reduced stress.

Some health factors we can't control, but we can choose good habits. I know firsthand that such choices take willpower and discipline *every day*. In addition, God has given us the medical technology to enhance our health. Let's use that too.

I often say to Jim, "I'm going to live to be 100 years old!" I know I'm not in total control of the length of my life, but I can be doing my part to live as long as God intends. And if I'm going to live to an old age, I want to be as healthy as possible!

I think of the little old man who was being interviewed on his 90th birthday. When asked how it felt to be that old, he replied, "Well, if I'd known I was going to get so old, I'd have taken better care of myself when I was young!"

Let's take good care of ourselves. We're worth it!

11
It's Not Just Your Imagination

It isn't your imagination. The world *is* out to get you. Your life really *is* out of control. Your husband and children *do* hate you. Your mother *did* mean that nasty remark she made last week. Your boss *does* think you're incompetent.

There, now. Feel better? Of course not. You were hoping none of it was true. But lately you no longer can tell what is truth and what is fiction.

Ruth, who was 51, was sure she was going crazy. Either that, or her whole world was falling apart. She and her husband had just had another terrible fight. He had left for work, angry at her as he'd been most mornings lately. They would get into arguments before she even knew what was happening.

Ron always blamed Ruth for the conflict. And he had

174

begun to say things like, "I can't take this any more. I'm not going to keep living like this for the rest of my life. I want something better than this." Ruth was scared he was thinking of a divorce.

But they were Christians! Divorce was unthinkable. They had married for life. Besides, she loved Ron with all her heart. She would be devastated without him.

In their 28 years of marriage Ruth and Ron had never had so much conflict. Ruth couldn't really grasp what was going on. She tried to reason with herself, but her perceptions about what was true in her world kept bouncing up and down.

She did know she felt horribly anxious and insecure much of the time. For the first time in her adult life, all kinds of worries and fears overwhelmed her. She tried keeping her focus on interests outside herself, but that didn't work.

Although she had many trouble spots, her biggest problem was Ron. In fact, she was scared about Ron's commitment to their marriage. His reasons for working late seemed very flimsy, and she wondered if he—like other men she had heard about—were having an affair.

She didn't want to accuse him if it weren't true. But her suspicions kept growing until her stomach was in knots. She felt jittery all over. A friend told her she looked like a "nervous wreck." She just had to ask him.

When they were both home one evening, she got up her courage to talk to him about it. As soon as she mentioned the subject, he blew up all over the place. She had never seen him so furious. He accused her of being petty and jealous. Soon they were sidetracked with charges and countercharges at each other. They never did resolve the original problem, and they went to bed feeling cold and stiff toward each other.

All night long Ruth was awake, not sure whether Ron's anger was because she hadn't trusted him or because he really was involved with someone else. And those awful anxieties still gnawed inside her.

She would look at him one time and decide, "Of course, he's really working all those extra hours. He may not be totally happy with me, but he would never get romantically involved with another woman."

Another time she would study him and think, "He just isn't himself. He seems so distant. When he talks, he is guarded and defensive. He loses his temper when I least anticipate it. He doesn't show me any affection. I wonder who *is* getting his love and attention?" And her mind would start rehearsing all the incidents and remarks that pointed to an affair.

Her thoughts plagued her, never leaving her alone and never getting better. . She felt like she was sliding down into a deep, narrow, frightfully black pit, and she'd never get out. She decided she had lost her mind along with Ron's love.

RECOGNIZE ANYONE?

As you may have guessed, Ruth is not a real person. (Or maybe you thought for sure I was talking about *you*.) Ruth is actually a compilation of what many women have described to me.

You may not suspect your husband of having an affair, but you may be having conflict with adult children, employers, employees, your pastor, a best friend, or a check-out clerk. Menopausal women tell me they are beset with doubts, hurt feelings, and uncontrollable crying spells more than ever before in their lives. They feel sad or anxious for no apparent reason. Or, the slightest little wrong sets off an uncharacteristic rage.

They can't stand crowds. They can't stand being alone. They no longer can pull off entertaining guests without falling apart. They dread the work they used to enjoy.

Joanne is such a woman. A 49-year-old single woman, she had been with the same firm for nearly 30 years. As the only secretary when the company first began, she had grown with the firm. She now did the work of a vice-president of an entire department, but she only had the title of assistant. She supervised many employees and actually was the brains of the operation. Her staff loved and respected her.

In restructuring workloads to fit their growth, her company brought in a young, inexperienced college graduate as vice-president. Joanne was still classified as an assistant. The new vice-president not only had the title, but also received a much higher salary because "he had a wife to support."

Joanne had been having menopausal symptoms, but— prior to the arrival of the vice-president—she was happy with her life and was keeping her health problems in place. She survived the blow of being ignored for the vice-presidential position. She even overlooked the salary difference. But when it became apparent that she had to do the vice-president's work and make up for his many mistakes, her hot flashes grew worse. She couldn't sleep and her body ached all over. Her emotions were almost more than she could handle.

This competent, gracious woman couldn't decide if the new situation was as bad as it seemed or if she were just imagining it. Every day she wrestled with maintaining a good attitude. She had successfully faced tough circumstances in earlier years, but this came at a time when her body and emotions complicated the work situation. After some months she left the company.

Women at menopause report that their emotions are like roller coasters—and much less dependable. Is this because they don't have enough to think about? Or are they simply giving in to themselves because menopause is supposed to be rough?

Some people think so. Many women who have had an easy passage or who haven't yet experienced menopause— and men who never will—are convinced it's all in a woman's head.

A few years ago a doctor in his 60s came to talk with me after I had spoken to a group of Christian men and women about changes at mid-life. I had briefly mentioned that menopause can be one of the stresses during this stage of life. After making a few general, complimentary remarks to me, the doctor drew me aside. In a harsh whisper that sounded like he was delivering a stern pronouncement as well as sharing a secret, he declared, "It's been my observation, over the many years of my practice, that the woman who has a difficult time at menopause is the woman who *expects* to have a difficult time."

"Oh, boy!" I thought. "Am I glad I'm not your patient! Or your wife."

EXAGGERATED AILMENTS

Sometime around age 50 I began to ache all over. I had always had some aches and pains, but my bones, muscles, and joints now hurt so much I could hardly concentrate on anything else. When I told my family doctor, he said, "What else can you expect at your age?" Later I complained about it to another family practice physician and two gynecologists. None of them gave any help except to suggest large doses of aspirin and ibuprofen.

Finally I made an appointment with our orthopedist. He had cared for several broken bones and other orthopedic problems in our family, and I felt he was a friend. Maybe *he* could get to the bottom of the problem. He ordered blood tests to check for arthritis and rheumatism. The results were negative.

Not knowing what to do next, I decided that—with the help of aspirin, vitamins, and prayer—I'd simply have to live with it. I didn't like taking a bunch of pills, but without them the pain was unbearable.

At times, thinking that the problem must be psychological weakness, I'd try going without the aspirin. Soon I'd be hurting so much, I could think of nothing else besides myself and my poor body. I was too busy to waste time that way. So I'd go back to the aspirin.

At the same time I was also having the tingling sensation throughout my body. When doctors couldn't find the source of that problem either, I really thought I was imagining things. I was afraid my husband and others thought so too.

Then I started having hot flashes. One day I had a grand one right in front of my gynecologist. He immediately prescribed estrogen. Not only did my hot flashes stop, my aches and pains diminished, and the tingling subsided.

Not one doctor ever told me a lack of estrogen might be the cause of my joint and muscle pain and tingling skin. But as I have researched this book and monitored my own reactions to different dosages of estrogen for more than five years, I have learned that estrogen—or the lack of it—can be closely related to many menopausal ailments.

This is not to say that estrogen is the answer for every health problem. Not at all! You need to find a good doctor with whom you feel comfortable and describe your complaints. But be well informed so that you can intelligently discuss your symptoms and the follow-up treatment. Be sure to remind him or her that you are menopausal age and ask if estrogen deprivation could be contributing to your symptoms.

Don't let anyone make you feel that your physical problems are only in your mind. Yes, your attitudes do influence how well you manage illness and pain, but your symptoms are real and someone needs to help you find relief. The next chapter will help you choose a doctor and ask the right questions.

YOU'RE TO BLAME

We probably travel on the biggest guilt trip when our mind and emotions are in pain and confusion. Somehow we are made to feel we should be able to control these and are more ashamed to get help when we need it.

Again, I admit that we do make choices that affect what our mind thinks and how we perceive life, and we can often exercise control over our emotional reactions. We also influence our physical health by what we eat and drink, how we rest, how much we exercise, and whether we get medical treatment when we need it.

However, some things happen in both our bodies and our psyches over which we have no control. It seems we feel that emotional distresses are more directly our fault than are physical ones. But, as one woman wrote on her questionnaire, "Menopausal symptoms are like the flu. They aren't your fault."

Some women do experience so much psychological trauma during menopause they need to be hospitalized. I have personally known some of them, and they were emotionally stable beforehand. They had some personality traits or thinking patterns that became unhealthy for a time, but they were "normal" people who temporarily came apart.

Many are well-educated, fulfilled professional women; some are well-educated, fulfilled homemakers. One professional singer and public relations consultant underwent "a mental breakdown brought on by a hysterectomy" 10 months earlier. She called it a "nightmarish slide into suicidal depression" because of the sudden change in hormones when her ovaries were removed.[1]

These women who are hospitalized or under psychiatric care should be applauded for getting help. They will probably get the medical attention they need to balance their hormones and become emotionally stable again.

BELIEVE IN YOU

The things you are experiencing aren't just your imagination. In addition to causing hot flashes, your hypothalamus and estrogen level affect your emotions. Although hot flashes are more measurable and definable than your gyrating emotions, you aren't crazy just because your feelings are topsy-turvy. Yes, long-standing problems and habits will play a part in your behavior now, but believe in yourself. Remember what you were like before menopause.

The very first time I asked my gynecologist if I could be experiencing an early menopause because my emotions were so out of control, he kept insisting I must have a psychological problem. He said I was too young for menopause.

I maintained that I had lived with myself for almost 40 years and that I had become increasingly observant of my physical and emotional states for the last 20. I had never before experienced such intense depression, anxiety, or anger. It wasn't that I hadn't encountered pain in the last four decades. With God's help, I had successfully handled *many* difficult times in life.

So I knew something had changed. It wasn't my circumstances. Something new was going on inside. As I've told you, I later learned that I probably was experiencing a decline in estrogen, which subsequently leveled out for a few more years.

After living with yourself this long, you can trust that you know some things about yourself. Maybe you do need some counseling help. This is nothing to be ashamed of. Most of us aren't embarrassed to look for help with physical problems, so let's get over our reluctance to admit our need for help with emotional problems.

Lois, 47, lives in a small town in Ohio. For over twenty years she has cared for her handicapped son along with trying to provide a normal life for her husband and two daughters. Four years ago her mother moved to a nursing home in their town so that Lois could visit her often and help care for her. At about the same time one of her daughters became very rebellious. Lois handled all the extra stress without much trouble. In fact, she was the traditional "pillar of strength" for the family.

About a year ago, however, she suddenly could take it no longer. She began to resent everyone's demands. No part of her life was ever her own. She was always tired. She became depressed and cried a lot.

Her husband, Roy, found her new behaviors to be very annoying and told her to "snap out of it!" He, according to Lois, didn't do much to help with the load. When she told him she thought she should see a doctor, he told her she just wanted sympathy.

"I knew something was going on," Lois told me. "I never had complained about all I had to do to help our son every day all those years. I didn't even look at it as drudgery. Now, I not only felt angry at him, I was upset with everyone else. Or else I'd be depressed for days. It sure didn't help any to have Roy think I was just being weak."

Lois began having heavy bleeding with her periods. When

she went to a doctor for that, she told him about her emotional changes. He immediately suggested she could be starting menopause and prescribed estrogen.

"I can't believe the difference!" Lois said. "Even Roy says it's good to have the old Lois back."

EVERYDAY LIVING

Some researchers, psychologists, and sociologists emphasize that menopause may be more difficult for some women because they are dealing with some trauma, such as divorce or the death of a parent, at the same time. But I find that many women don't face such drastic circumstances; they simply have trouble coping with the ordinary daily stresses. They have carried on busy lives for many years, but now they get nervous when too much is happening at once. They readily coped with difficulties in the past, but when something goes wrong now, their emotions—and some-times their behaviors—go out of control. They misplace things and drive themselves silly looking for them. They forget where they are going, and if they get there, they can't remember what they came for.

Marla told me that she used to find herself driving along in her car and suddenly not know where she was going. She couldn't remember if she were going to or from something. She would pull over beside the street to try to think. If it didn't come to her, she would go home until she could recall what she was supposed to be doing. You can imagine how this would drive you crazy! After she was put on hormone replacement therapy for other reasons, her memory improved and she no longer forgot where she was going.

UNFAIR

Menopausal women often are surprised to find themselves full of self-pity. They have given and served and turned the other cheek for decades; now they feel abused and exploited. They wonder when they will receive bouquets like they've been giving to others all these years. Who even appreciates all they have done for everybody? And who ever does anything for them?

Then, adding insult to injury, everything about their body is sagging and bagging. They look and feel *old*. To top it off, their gray-haired and portly husband is considered mature and dignified. A man's wrinkles mean he's experienced and wise; a woman's wrinkles mean she's a haggard has-been. Or, as a little quip in *Better Homes and Gardens* says, "Women will never be the equal of men until they can have large bald spots and think they're good-looking."[2]

Of course, I know some women don't let their aging affect them. I admire the ones who are secure enough about themselves that they graciously accept their creases, gray hair, old age spots, stooping shoulders, and errant waistlines. But I wonder if even they don't have their secret times of lamentation.

WHO AM I?

Self-esteem comes under attack at menopause for many reasons. Not only is the aging process tearing at the image a woman has of herself, but her role as mother has changed so that she is less needed and—she feels—less wanted. If she is trying to reenter the job market or enter for the first time, she may face subtle, if not open, discrimination.

When she goes to shop for clothes, she finds that the styles are either for the young and slim or for matrons like her mother. Even the classes and special programs at her church cater to the young or the very old. She knows in her heart that she is still a valuable person, but when it looks as if the world doesn't recognize that, she questions it herself.

I recently met Ginny, a 46-year-old professional woman, who learned I was writing this book on menopause. After she said she really wanted to read it when it was published, she said, "I haven't gone through menopause yet, but I'll be glad when I do because then I'll *finally find out who I am.*"

At first I gulped and wanted to say, "Oh, Ginny, if you only knew what may be ahead!" I thought of telling her that probably menopause, for a time, would destroy what little handle she presently had on her identity and worth. But I caught myself and, in the little time we had together, I gently told her about a few of the changes she could expect, not only in her body, but also in her roles and relationships.

I didn't tell her that menopause could cause her to be less sure of herself than she is now. I didn't want to dump too much on her, nor did I want to sound as if I see only the negative side of menopause. I don't think that all menopausal women will experience only bad things at all times.

HELP!

I have, however, heard and read and personally encountered enough difficulties at this time of life to know that a majority of women would like some help. Women in the thick of it need empathy and aid; younger women need to get prepared.

Premenopausal women seem to fall into two categories: women who are terrified of menopause and women who are ignorant of it. Perhaps I should add a third—women who have tried to find out about menopause from their doctors and have been told very little or nothing.

When Ginny asked her doctor how she'd know when she was in menopause, all he would tell her was, "When you have hot flashes." She decided the reason he didn't give her much information was because he didn't know much about menopause.

To get a driver's license in any state, we have to read that state's handbook on the rules of the road and pass a test. To get married, we needed to get a blood test and a marriage license. Some of us got premarital counseling. Before we had our babies, most of us read at least one book on child care. We probably did some reading and preparing to get ready for menstruation. Let's do the same for menopause!

Support groups are now popular for all kinds of situations—alcohol and drug addiction, overeating, divorce recovery, single parenting, sexual abuse, and many others. Our church has all these, plus groups for parents who have lost children in death, people who must care for aging parents, couples with infertility problems, blended families, and even wives whose husbands have had an affair. Let's have one for menopause!

In recent decades, parents of teenagers have found comfort in knowing that their children aren't abnormal when their moods are up and down and when their attempts at independence sometimes cause pain for everyone. By reading, talking with other parents, and attending discussion groups about normal teen development, parents have learned that other adolescents are similar to theirs. To understand normal teen behavior helps parents ride the stormy adolescent waves, knowing that calm *will come*.

In the same way, if we share information about menopause, perhaps we can help women and their families more successfully navigate the stormy times. Perhaps we can eliminate the situations faced by Lois in this chapter and Marjorie in Chapter 1.

We aren't going crazy. Menopause symptoms aren't just our imagination and we don't need to feel guilty. We are normal. But we certainly could use some help!

PART III

SURVIVING
AND THRIVING

12

The Doctor Connection

"Doctors are only good at charging. They could not care less if they help you!" wrote one woman on her questionnaire. My study of menopausal women indicated that a total of 370 doctors had been consulted for help regarding menopause. Only 99 of these were perceived as helpful.

Remember that these responses were from women with menopause symptoms. Do these statistics mean these women were difficult to please? Their perceptions were awry? They don't know anything about their bodies and emotions after all these years? Or they were foolishly expecting miracles? I'm not sure what it all means, but it certainly indicates dissatisfaction.

Most of my good doctor friends would be the first to tell you that their profession has its share of disinterested, greedy, overworked, and even dishonest practitioners. Many are incompetent, or untrained, specifically in the field of menopause.

Probably in your profession or in that of your husband there are also some inept, disagreeable, and insincere folks. We don't, however, condemn the entire profession for the sins of a few. We still send our children to school, even though some teachers are inept. We put our money in banks, although some bank employees have been known to embezzle. We buy groceries, clothes, and gasoline from companies that misrepresent their products or provide poor service.

Instead of berating doctors, let's see what we can do to choose the one best for our needs, ask the right questions, and follow his or her suggested treatment.

HOW TO CHOOSE

Your choice, of course, depends a great deal on where you live. It also may depend on your medical coverage and whether you get to choose your own doctor. If you live in a metropolitan area, you have many doctors from which to choose. That's not always an advantage, because you may wonder how to find a trustworthy one. If you live in a rural area, your choice is limited, and you may have to drive a distance.

You may have been seeing good, old Dr. Faithful for the last 30 years. In fact, he delivered all your babies and just delivered your first grandchild. He has stitched all your kids and nursed your husband through his prostatitis. But he may not be aware of the latest research on menopause. He may do little to help you, and he even may cause you to feel you're just imagining things.

If you live in a sparsely populated area, you probably think you'll cause a scandal if you change doctors. Everyone will know about it. And besides, Dr. and Mrs. Faithful are in your church every Sunday, and you're afraid you couldn't look them in the eye.

Remember, it's your body, and you're going to have to live with it the rest of your life, perhaps long after dear Dr. Faithful is dead. Also, notice that wise, old Dr. Faithful patronizes the businesses and professions that best meet his needs. You don't have to be rude, but do be courageous enough to get the best care for yourself.

Or you may have moved recently and feel at a loss about selecting a new doctor. Start with the people you know who are most likely to have seen a doctor for the same symptoms. Then ask your pastor, pastor's wife, church secretary, president of the women's fellowship, and/or your neighbors. Call your county medical association or local hospital referral service for recommendations.

Get out your telephone directory. Turn to the *physicians* section. Look under *gynecologist*. You may need to look under *obstetrician/gynecologist*. If you can, avoid the ones who advertise "infertility" as one of their specialties. They're probably not seeing many menopausal women!

I suggest a gynecologist whose practice includes a good number of women your age. An obstetrician/gynecologist may be almost solely devoted to young women in the baby-delivering era of life.

Obstetricians, of course, know about menopause in

biological ways that we do not; however, they may not be keeping up with the latest menopausal research. Many family practitioners are also very knowledgeable about the subject; others are not. You need to find out what is each particular doctor's area of interest.

When you have settled on the doctor you would like to try, don't be afraid to ask several questions when you telephone the receptionist. If she seems too hurried to answer or gives you the feeling you aren't entitled to such information, say thank-you and wait to call at a later time or on another day. Perhaps you will get someone different or the original one will be in a different mood.

Remember that receptionists and nurses don't necessarily reflect the attitudes of the doctor. Sometimes good help is hard to find—or it's a bad day for everyone at the office. You do need your questions answered, though, before you agree to an appointment.

Your first question should always be, "Is the doctor taking any new patients?" If the doctor is not taking any new patients, you need to look for another doctor.

Even if a doctor has been recommended by another doctor or by your very best friend, you should ask about the doctor's qualifications. Here are some suggested questions:

1. Does the doctor have current medical board certification in his or her chosen field? (For example, the American College of Obstetrics/Gynecology or the American Board of Family Practitioners.)
2. How long has the doctor been in practice?
3. At which hospitals is the doctor on staff?
4. What percentage of the doctor's practice is made up

of menopausal women? (Or whatever medical specialty you need.)

5. Does the doctor shave, brush his or her teeth, and use
deodorant? (Oops! Just kidding!)
Then you'll want to ask additional questions:

6. What are the charges for each office call? What other
charges should I expect? When is payment expected?
Who fills out insurance forms?

7. What is likely to happen on my first visit? Should I be
prepared for blood or urine tests?

8. Is there anything else I need to know about becoming
a patient?

You might feel more comfortable if the board-certified
gynecologist or other practitioner you select has been in
practice a long time, but don't forget that sometimes young
doctors know the latest research. Make sure you choose a
doctor on the staff of a reputable hospital you would want to
use if you needed to.

If you feel satisfied that this is the doctor you would like
to consult, make an appointment. On your first visit, arrive a
little early with an optimistic attitude. Take along a list of the
questions you want to ask so that you don't waste your
doctor's time or forget something important.

YOU'RE PART OF THE TEAM

Gone are the days when we expected doctors to be gods.
Well, we still want them to perform miracles, but we now
question their decisions more often! In the past, we

obediently swallowed any pill or liquid they prescribed, meekly submitted to every test, and didn't very often doubt their judgment. After all, they had a medical education, and we were just ignorant peons. Some doctors cultivated that atmosphere, but many times we didn't know we could participate in the decisions.

This was very clear one time when I talked to an older women I'll call Ethel. She had gone through extensive tests for a number of complaints, and I was trying to learn from her what the doctor had discovered and what her various pills were to do for her. She wasn't sure what the diagnosis was, but the doctor had prescribed three different medicines.

Ethel was starting to experience dizziness since she had seen the doctor, and I wondered if one of the medications might be the cause. When I pressed her for the names of her pills, she replied, "Well, I don't know, but the *doctor* gave them to me." She said the word "doctor" with that hallowed tone of voice that implied the pills had to be all right if *he* prescribed them.

Today most doctors are glad that we want to be actively involved in our health care. They are pleased when we are informed and know how to ask intelligent questions. They want us to know what medications we are taking and why, and they want to be told if a treatment isn't working.

If your doctor is threatened by your participation, consider two possibilities:

1. Your manner is inappropriate. You may be coming across as arrogant or as a "crabby old biddy."
2. You may need a different doctor.

I changed doctors a few years ago because the one I was

seeing became hostile when I suggested that a different form of estrogen replacement might be more effective. (I'm sure *my* attitude wasn't wrong, or I wouldn't be telling you about it!)

He was a young general practitioner to whom I had first gone when I had the flu. When he seemed interested in helping me with menopause symptoms, I decided to go under his care. After a time, however, I began to feel uneasy about his treatment plan.

I had been doing some studying about the management of postmenopausal symptoms and ERT specifically. I also had my past experience with other doctors as a standard. Since I felt my response to the particular therapy he was using was poor, I wanted to discuss an alternative method.

He became very defensive and asked, "Are you challenging my judgment?"

Although I often am intimidated by authority figures, this time I replied, "No, not exactly, but I wonder if another form of ERT might work better."

"Well, I've treated hundreds of women with this method. I know what I'm doing!" he said.

I then asked, "Doctor, do you also practice at another facility?"

He said that he did not. I said no more, but silently told myself this was my last visit. I had been in his waiting room at various times of the day every three weeks for four months, and I never had seen even one other woman my age! Those "hundreds of women" didn't seem to be visible. I lost my confidence in him.

PATIENTLY PERSISTENT

"If at first you don't succeed, try, try, try again," is a useful motto when it comes to finding a doctor who is right for you. Many women get discouraged about finding a good doctor or feel embarrassed to admit they aren't satisfied. Doctors aren't perfect. (Neither are their patients!) But if you feel you aren't getting competent care, you must be brave enough to look until you do.

In addition to good care, it's nice to have friendliness and empathy from a doctor. However, not every person with the intelligence, technical abilities, and ambition to get through medical school has good social skills. If I had to choose between a doctor having rapport or having expertise, I guess I'd pick the one with skill. But I'm more comfortable when a doctor has both.

I kept looking until I found one who is both capable and amiable. On top of that, my doctor is a woman! My age! Her specialty is gynecology. A very attractive woman, she also has the same spiritual values I do. She sounds almost too good to be true, but everyone I refer to her agrees she's just what we've all been looking for.

Patience and persistence are also helpful when you are working with a doctor on a particular treatment program. The two of you may have to try several times to find the right medication, adjust the dosage, combat allergies, or whatever.

Don't give up. Often many different combinations of treatments can be used. For example, if one type of estrogen or progesterone causes a bad reaction or doesn't create a strong enough response, let your doctor know. Don't simply decide that doctors don't know what they're doing, or that your case is hopeless.

UNDERSTANDING THE DOCTOR

Sometimes we are pretty critical of doctors. We often categorize them as rich, self-important, uncaring creatures. However, I know many who are very, very human. They do care very much about their patients. In spite of their professional training, many of them grieve when a patient dies. They "worry" when a treatment isn't working. They agonize over a hard decision that must be made for the patient's good.

Many of them are very humble servants. They *are* busy, however. You might be amazed at the number of patients they have to see in an hour—not just so they can get more money, but because the demand for their help is great. So if they seem in a hurry, try to understand. You are, however, entitled to a fair amount of time, so make sure you get it.

I also know doctors who aren't rich. Most of us can't begin to imagine what their education has cost them and the cost of setting up an office with minimum accommodations. Many are in debt for years. In addition, today's malpractice insurance rates are unbelievable. I am aware of doctors who have had to take out loans to meet their staff payroll.

Some doctors have deliberately chosen to keep their practice small so that they have time to be a husband and father. Thus, there's no doctor's house in a doctors' neighborhood for them. On the other hand, you, too, aren't made of money, so you need to use your medical dollars wisely and get the best advice and treatment possible.

IN THE DOCTOR'S SHOES

It also helps to see the difference between the doctor's goals and yours when it comes to medical care. The authors of *Midlife Health* remind us:

> Doctors have been trained to identify and treat disease. Surgeons in particular see their role as identifying and removing disease. Meanwhile, you, as a patient, want a sympathetic ear, and safe, effective, and easy cures. . . .
>
> The problem is that the doctors see their role as being either identifying or "ruling out" known disease, while [the patient] sees their job as alleviating her pain, preferably without major surgery. . . . Doctors have a tendency to say "there's nothing wrong with you" when what they really mean is that "using currently available tests, I cannot identify any known disease that explains your problem." Patients, used to miracle cures, do not always accept that the same medical profession that can do heart-lung transplants cannot cure an arthritis pain.[1]

Another point to remember is that the sheer amount of new information on any medical topic is staggering. When we say that a doctor isn't keeping up-to-date, we need to be mindful that it is humanly impossible to know the latest on every medical subject. Doctors are required to attend a certain number of educational seminars a year to maintain certification in their chosen field, but even then, it's hard to keep up on all the current data.

The amount of technical literature that comes across their desks would blow us away. But we want them to read and digest it all. At the same time, we want them to give us extra minutes during our appointments, do their surgeries competently, make their hospital rounds leisurely, keep their records thoroughly, and be good to their families.

WHEN TO SEE A DOCTOR

To some of you, it may seem silly to even talk about when it's important to get a doctor's help. But I've found that many women try to ignore menopausal symptoms or other important health problems. They're either frightened by old wives' tales or think no doctor understands. Sometimes they don't want anyone to think they aren't strong, or they don't realize the consequences of not getting help, or they're afraid they'll learn they have an awful disease.

It's impossible to list every circumstance for which you need a doctor's help, but as little thought-prodders, the following suggestions are a start. You should see a doctor if:

- you're having hot flashes, and you're in the high-risk category for osteoporosis.
- you're having heart palpitations, prolonged insomnia, extreme irritability, tingling skin, or painful joints.
- you have vaginal dryness, urinary leakage, itching, or burning.
- your emotions are unexplainably off-balance.
- you have excessive or irregular vaginal bleeding.
- you find breast lumps or have a discharge from your nipples.

- you are chronically tired after sufficient rest.
- it's time for your annual physical. Don't put it off! Every woman over 30 needs a yearly physical exam.

ASKING THE RIGHT QUESTIONS

Again, it's not possible to presume to know all the questions you need to ask your doctor. I simply want to assure you that you have the right to ask questions.

First of all, know as much about yourself and your problem as possible. If you need to, keep a diary of your symptoms so you can report accurately to your doctor. Read and study about your symptoms so that you are a knowledgeable participant in your own health care. Make a list of what you want to ask your doctor.

When you go for your appointment, use your diary and the list of questions. Have your list organized by category and items of importance ahead of time, so that you get the best use of your minutes with the doctor.

Let the nurse attending you know that you have certain questions for the doctor. Tell the doctor right away too. Don't wait until the doctor's ready to go out the door and then try to flag him or her down with your list.

When the doctor suggests a certain medication or procedure, keep asking questions until you know enough to feel comfortable. Don't let the medical jargon scare you off. Ask the doctor to give it to you in terms you can understand and remember. If you need to, write things down on your paper with your list of questions.

If your doctor suggests surgery, adapt the questions we

suggested in Chapter 7 regarding a hysterectomy. Tell your doctor that you will be seeking a second opinion. If he or she is a true professional, he or she won't be insulted. Get at least one other opinion from a doctor who is not in the same medical group nor a referral from the first doctor.

FOLLOW INSTRUCTIONS

After you leave the doctor's office, be sure you get full value for your investment of time and money—do what the doctor recommends. Get the prescriptions filled and take them as directed. Carry through with any other outlined procedures.

If you aren't sure about something, call the doctor's nurse. Often the nurse can clarify a minor point or will ask the doctor and call you back. Don't just let the matter slide and not take complete care of yourself.

HAPPILY EVER AFTER

You have a right to expect certain things from your doctor: expertise, courtesy, understanding, honesty, confidentiality, to name a few. Your doctor also needs certain things from you: courtesy, honesty, cooperation, and prompt payment for services.

I hope you don't feel like the woman at the beginning of this chapter—that your doctor only wants your money. Most of them genuinely do want to help. Today there are much easier ways to get rich than to be a doctor, so adjust your attitude and expect your doctor to have your best health in mind.

13
A Place for You

"It's difficult for me to realize that I'm not the same as I used to be—and never will be the same again," one 58-year-old midwestern woman wrote on her survey.

Never being the same again is probably one of the biggest sources of grief for many of us. We aren't accustomed to the way we are now; we liked our lives much better before. Those were the good, old days when—as we remember it—we had ourselves, our families, and perhaps our careers under better control.

THE GOOD YOUNG DAYS

We grieve partly because we feel we didn't fully appreciate our circumstances then. I personally regret that I didn't value my physical body more when it was slim and firm. I

204

always concentrated on the flaws. My bust was too small. My hips were too wide for the rest of me. It was hard to stand straight. For many years I was actually *too* skinny.

When I look at pictures of myself from those days now, I realize that I had a better than average figure, and my face wasn't bad either. At least, it was unwrinkled. I didn't comprehend then how wonderful it was to have resilient skin around my eyes. Putting eye makeup on my spongy skin now is as tricky as applying eyeliner on rising bread dough!

I occasionally tell my three daughters who are in their twenties and thirties, "Be sure to enjoy your body while it's young!"

I also tell myself, "Be sure to enjoy *your* body as it is now, because when you are 80, you're going to think your 55-year-old body was great."

STRETCHING TO FIT

This time in our lives is like wearing a new pair of high-heeled shoes we bought on sale. Although the shoes are too narrow, the color goes great with our best dress. When we wear them, no one knows how those shoes pinch our feet and make us feel miserable all over! We just keep smiling and going on . . . until our feet hurt so badly we no longer can take another step. As we hobble to a seat and kick off the shoes, anyone who notices thinks we are silly or unsophisticated. Until those shoes are broken in by our feet or stretched by a shoemaker, they are going to be uncomfortable.

At menopause life all around us is changing. The new life

will feel uncomfortable until we get used to it. We may need professional help—at least, a medical doctor, and perhaps a counselor—to assist in our adjustment. It will take some time to get used to our new territory.

During the time that I was entering menopause, Jim and I made a career change. We went from being pastor and wife of a large, active, evangelical, midwestern church to being professor and adjunct instructor in a California theological seminary, along with founding Mid-Life Dimensions. After five years the work with this organization had increased so much, we felt it necessary to resign from teaching and devote ourselves fully to mid-life concerns.

REDRAWING THE LINES

Because we generally lecture together at seminars, co-direct the office ministry, and work in offices a few feet apart, we are with each other all day every day. Our evenings are also spent together. When we aren't traveling, we both are busy at our desks until the secretaries leave, and sometimes long after. That usually means that I haven't done much dinner preparation. On top of that, I'm bone tired. Jim pitches in with meals and cleanup. Sometimes he graciously does it all.

As you can imagine, that's a big change from when he was pastoring a church. Even though I was very much a part of the ministry, I was not at the office with him and I did not attend all the meetings he did. I didn't stand with him to preach. Neither did he accompany me in my daily sphere of activities nor do my housework.

Even though I greatly appreciate our sharing of household tasks now, we have had to talk about the boundaries. I began to feel frustrated and unfulfilled when I went very long without cooking, or grocery shopping (after I got through that stage when I didn't want to shop alone). On occasions when Jim did the laundry, I could hardly keep my hands off. Some jobs just seemed like my domain.

What we really had to talk over was cooking Thanksgiving dinner. Jim had gradually taken over the turkey preparations. Then he began making the dressing, using his recipe instead of mine. One year he decided he'd like to bake the pies—not just one kind, but three different kinds. Well, I still had my special sweet potato dish to make, until the year he wanted to take on that job too!

I suddenly realized that much of my enjoyment of Thanksgiving was getting robbed by a very well-meaning husband. I certainly didn't have time to do it all, but for my own soul's sake, I needed to retain parts of the task. Once I told Jim my feelings, he very gladly agreed on a comfortable split of the dinner preparations.

NEW DAYS

Because we postmenopausal women are, more than ever before, a generation busy with careers, we're still carving out our roles and expectations. Sometimes even our family has to get rid of their stereotypes about women our age.

I thought you might chuckle over this poem I found in my mother's letter drawer. It had been sent to her from her sister at the time she had gone back to teaching after many years of child rearing.

THE VERSATILE AGE

The old rocking chair is empty today
Grandma is no longer in it.
She is off in her car to her office or shop
And buzzes around every minute.
No one shelves Grandma back on the shelf;
She is versatile, forceful, dynamic.
That is not a pie in the oven, my dear,
Her baking today is ceramic!
You won't see her trundling off early to bed
From her place in a warm chimney nook.
Her typewriter clickety-clacks through the night
For Grandma is writing a book.
Grandma ne'er takes a backward look
To slow her steady advancing.
She won't tend the babies for you any more
For Grandma is taking up dancing.
She is not content with crumbs of old thoughts
With meager and second-hand knowledge.
Don't bring your mending for Grandma to do
For Grandma has gone back to college.

—Anonymous

You'll notice that the poem was written before the computer age had taken hold: today's grandmas use word processors instead of typewriters.

NO SPOT TO FILL

Many postmenopausal women feel that their life doesn't have much to offer. For many reasons it looks to these women like everyone else is having the good time.

Elizabeth is typical of many women who have shared with me their bleak outlook. For nearly 30 years she has given herself to her children and her husband. She has had other interests, but those don't look very important or stimulating now. No one gives her credit for doing much else other than mothering. (As if this weren't a gigantic enough job!)

Elizabeth's husband has gone back to graduate school to advance his career. Her children are in college and doing well. Everyone is doing something exciting—except her. On top of that, they are living in a new community where no one even recognizes her for her husband's position, let alone hers.

She summed it all up when she said, "There's just *no place* for me."

I've known Elizabeth for years, and she's no whiner. She's usually an outgoing person with lots of sparkle. But menopause—the change of life—is approaching when so many other parts of her life are also changing.

The *change of life* takes away our fertility at the same time that other very important roles in our lives seem to be vanishing. Our children are independent and choosing their own paths. They may be starting their families, which rightfully become more important to them than their parental family. We shift from being actively needed to being consulted—irregularly.

When the kids were at home, we may have complained

about all the coming and going. Now, even though we may be active with our own interests, we ache inside for the noise and the happy commotion. We liked being included in all that vim and vigor. Now evenings are too quiet.

With the nest demanding less time now, women are free to consider where else to use their time. Many women tell me that they have never really had a career other than mothering and homemaking. Perhaps they took clerical, waitressing, or similar positions as a way to earn some money, but these weren't actually professions to them. Now what are they supposed to do?

They may feel they don't have the time, money, or brains to go to school or to get training for something they'd really like to do. Who'd want an old lady, anyway?

Lots of people would. When we need new staff at Mid-Life Dimensions, we always advertise for older, "mature" women. Our young assistants are good, but the more life experience a woman has, the more she can just naturally empathize with the hurting people who contact us. This isn't something that can be taught. It comes from living.

Many professions need someone with all the experience you have had in managing a household and family. If you haven't been a wife or a mother, you still have gained wisdom and insight from what you've been doing all these years. Start adding it up, writing it down, and giving your jobs and activities titles and job descriptions as if they had been accumulating on a career vita sheet.

AT THE BEGINNING

Actually, you may need to start with your self-esteem. If you think you are of little value, you will have trouble seeing where you fit with family, job, and the rest of the world. I have found it helpful to use what I call "The Three A's"— Assess, Accept, Appreciate.

Assess

First of all, take an inventory of who you are and what you have to offer to everyone important to you. Make at least four lists.

Write at the top of one: "*My Strengths and Abilities.*" Focus on your positive personality traits, your education, the things you are equipped to do because of your background and experiences.

Title another sheet of paper: "*Things I Like to Do.*" These can be anything from the serious to the silly. Consider every area of life. What do you really like to do? (Take a quick check of how many of these activities you actually *get* to do—you may find you are starving your inner self.)

Make another list: "*What I Want to Accomplish Before I Die.*" Nothing got me started on this list faster than the time I thought I had breast cancer. My mind rushed ahead to speculate what I wanted to get done if I were to die in a few months. When the scare was over (the lump turned out to be nonmalignant, after all), I realized I still needed to decide what I want to accomplish before I die, even though I got a reprieve from breast cancer. How can I make the best use of the time I have? What and who are most important in the days I have left?

Still a fourth list could be, "*What I Have to Give.*" If you wonder if you're valuable to anyone, start listing the ways you are—or could be. Put names down one side of your paper and jot down what you can *do* and *be* to each one.

At a time in life when you may be feeling very insecure about your relationship with your husband, teen or adult children, or special friends, it will help if you know yourself and what you can offer to others. Instead of being afraid of their rejection, reach out to them—with sensitivity and with confidence—and give what you have and are.

As you contemplate all that you've written on your lists, you will begin to see that God didn't make a mistake when he made you. You are worthwhile! Keep adding to your lists every few days, and reread them whenever your spirits need a boost.

Accept

As you assess yourself, you will eventually think about your weaknesses too. Actually, you probably could make a longer list of these than of your strengths. Please don't. Be honest, but don't be too hard on yourself.

As you consider all that makes you *you*, come to terms with the parts you don't like. Change what you can and accept the rest. For instance, I am tall—the same height as my husband. I can't change that, but I can be at peace about it. Right now I am overweight. I *can* change that, and I'm working on it.

I grew up in a rural area and went to a small one-room school for eight years, then I went to a high-school of 100 students. We hardly had any library or science facilities, but we had teachers who cared that we learned what they could teach. I can't change my country background and don't want to. I accept it as part of what makes me who I am today. (Sometimes, driving down a twelve-lane Los Angeles freeway, I chuckle as I realize that at this moment I'm seeing more cars than I saw in all of my childhood years. No wonder I sometimes long for the wide, open spaces!)

I had parents who were sensitive and loving. I married Jim, who is gentle and insightful. He cares deeply for people. I, too, have developed a genuine concern for people and their problems. Sometimes that's very inconvenient, and it certainly isn't lucrative. But I can't walk away from it. That's who I am. That's my past and my present. And I accept it.

I also care for details. I want to know all about what's happening, or what someone is thinking and feeling, or what needs to be done. Wrongly used, that characteristic can get me into trouble. I could become a busybody. Rightly used, people get cared for and feel loved, and office details are handled accurately. I accept that I am a "detail" person and try to use it correctly.

Accepting yourself, your personality, your background, your experiences, your present circumstances—whatever you are working at accepting—is something that you must do yourself. It helps to get feedback from other people, especially if it's positive and not condemning, but you still must do the work of self-acceptance *yourself*.

Appreciate

Appreciate who you are. That doesn't mean you are proud. True humility is acknowledging that God made you what you are and gave you what you have. Recognizing your abilities and positive qualities makes you better balanced than if you're belittling yourself. To confidently know and use your strengths—while giving credit where credit is due— also gives more honor to your Creator than to criticize and demean yourself.

Remind yourself that you have been made in God's image. In addition, you know that what God makes is beautiful and good. Perhaps you'd like to recite this little poem to yourself frequently:

> Believe it,
> You are a real find,
> A joy in someone's heart.
> You're a jewel, unique and priceless.
> I don't care how you feel.
> Believe it,
> God don't make no junk.[1]
> —Herbert B. Barks, Jr.

Actually, once you come to accept and appreciate yourself, you are freer to do the same for others. When you can forgive your own faults and delight in how you are made, you will be more tolerant and appreciative of your family, friends, and co-workers.

NEXT STEP

Now that you've begun to assess, accept, and appreciate, you're ready for *action*! You're getting set to fill that place that's available for you. And that's what the next chapter is all about.

14
Setting Your Course

Menopause is not a disease. In and of itself, it is not fatal. You no longer need to feel like a victim—of menopause, of the people around you, or of life itself.

You may need to mourn the passing of an important era of life. This is all right to do for a while. Even after you think you've successfully moved on to the next stage, the grief may come back occasionally. That's okay too. That's normal. You're normal.

Women several years past menopause have hopeful words to pass on to the rest of us:

With patience and understanding, you will be yourself again.

I was out of it for more than two years. I didn't want to do anything and my mind just was not in gear. Now I'm normal again.

The biggest reassurance I had that the emotional changes I experienced weren't "all in my mind" or from a lack of coping skills [was] when they went away . . . they just left.

I was so bitchy—there's no other word for it—but now I'm doing fine. Everything else is the same, but I'm able to deal with it all again.

I am like a new woman. My husband thinks it's a miracle! We both praise God.

So, if you aren't quite victorious yet like these other women, what do you do? Remember to *assess*, *accept*, and *appreciate* yourself as we outlined in the last chapter. It's something to keep doing, and eventually you'll be strong enough for *action*.

START WITH "GOOD-BYE . . . HELLO"

You might want to arrange some sort of rite of passage for yourself. Perhaps you and your husband and children could have a special meal together, observing the end of one phase of life and the beginning of a new one. Or you and your husband might plan a sentimental trip together.

Maybe you would feel more comfortable spending time with your best friend or a small group of women. You may want to have a quiet time alone, officially recognizing your passage to this next stage of life.

You don't have to make a big deal out of it. It's your time. Be as public or as private as you wish. Whatever you decide to do, you will probably find that it helps bring closure to a very large section of your life. Then you can look forward to opening the pages of the chapter ahead.

Don't worry if you are months or years overdue with such

a rite of passage. It's better to do it now than never. I was a few years late in recognizing what a turning point my hysterectomy had been. One of the things I did was to buy a big black coffee mug that pronounces in large gold letters, "Over the hill and off the pill!"

Laugh. Cry. Stomp your feet a little if you need to. Then set your sights on what's important and get going.

ON YOUR MARK, GET SET, KNOW!

You've already started on a significant step by reading this book. Being informed gives you an edge on the whole ordeal. Oh, yes, you still have to go through it, but you should be able to do it in better health and spirits. You know more about making wise decisions—decisions that make a difference in how you feel now and how you'll feel in the future.

If the average woman studies and learns about menopause, perhaps we'll see a change in the osteoporosis statistics in a few years. Maybe fewer women will struggle with heart problems. I hope that more marriages will stay together that might have broken during menopause. All this, because our generation, and the ones to come, know more about how to handle the symptoms.

THEN GROW

Whatever your situation, you can find a way to grow. A growing woman is an interesting woman—to others and to herself. For a number of years I have been looking at what makes some elderly women a joy to be with and others a pain. What I notice over and over again is that the "nice" ones are fresh and growing, the "grumpy" ones have stagnated. The enjoyable ones see opportunity around every corner; the difficult ones think their life is over. I vow to be one of the fresh, growing ones!

Maybe you need to go back to school. It's never too late. Adult education classes, for credit or not for credit, are everywhere. Even if you don't use what you learn to earn money, you'll find the stimulation to be worth more than dollars.

It's not too late to launch into a career either. You probably have lots of vigorous, healthy years left. Even if you don't live a long time, you will be glad you got started. A good book to guide you is *What Color Is Your Parachute?* by Richard Bolles.[1]

Perhaps you just need to grow right where you are. You don't need to start a new career, new hobby, or go to school. You can just read, think, and discuss new ideas with other people. Turn your creative ideas loose on whatever you're doing now. Do things to deliberately break the old routine. Keep from falling into a rut and staying there.

This sounds like a lot of hype, doesn't it? Especially if this is a bad day—or month—or year—for you. That's all right. You can throw the book at the wall. I can't see you. Even if I could, it's still okay for you to be angry.

STRETCHING OUT

Eventually you'll come to a time when you're ready to move on. I've found that the most fulfilling thing I can do for myself is to make someone else happy. When I'm down, I get up lots faster if I think of something to do for somebody. Even if I think I don't have another minute in my day to tackle one more activity, I get rejuvenated if I take a jiffy to send a card, make a call, or do some little thing for someone.

You could also practice being more sensitive to the world around you. What are people feeling? Why do they feel that way? What is causing their behavior? How would you feel and act if you were in their shoes?

At the end of each day you could ask yourself some questions that would help you appreciate your experiences and stimulate your progress toward being a more interesting person. What new things have you learned today? What did you see that you've never seen before? What little joy did you experience? You may have to use more fertilizer, but you still can grow!

If you could talk to the women in my study, you'd hear them saying, "What has helped me most during menopause is to keep active." Then they'd list things like new hobbies, taking classes, being with people, and finding a fulfilling career.

One woman wrote, "Keep busy. Push yourself on the days you feel so blah, even if all you get done is the dishes. Just one thing done is an accomplishment worth being proud of."

Another confided, "Being needed is the most important part of my life. I'm in a mid-life career of real estate, and I have clients who wouldn't think of buying or selling without 'my expertise.' I'm taking one course per term, working on a Master's in Theology. My friends love to hear what I'm learning, and I'm glad to pass it on. I'm serving on. . . ." She went on listing committees and projects she's involved in, and ran out of space to write it all.

FRIENDLY FAMILY TIES

One of the biggest areas of your life is probably your family—your husband, children, parents, siblings. If you aren't married or don't have children, please think of your friends as family during this discussion.

Most of the women in my survey said their families were little or no help during menopause, and many said their families added to their problems. A few credited their husbands with being understanding, but almost all indicated their husbands were not. Mothers were practically useless, and children were a negative.

We won't go into all the family dynamics that can cause aloofness, heartaches, and misunderstandings today, but I'd like to give some suggestions for what you can do to *help your family help you* during menopause:

- *Be honest.* Tell them what you are feeling. Let them know you don't understand all that's happening to you. Warn them when you feel more upset than usual. Tell them—without unnecessary whining—about your physical symptoms.

- *Share the medical facts with them.* You don't have to give them the whole load at once, but do let them in on what health factors you're dealing with.

- *Be patient with them.* This may be the first time you haven't been the strong one. It might take some time for them to catch on that you need their help.

- *Be courteous.* This may be asking a lot, and you may not even realize you're not being kind—but try. I've known some women who take advantage of their situation and let the fur fly where it will. That's not going to encourage your family to be understanding of you.

- *Affirm their attempts to help you.* Your husband may think he's doing what you need by insisting you go shopping when you really just want to spend a few quiet hours with him. Thank him very much for his thoughtfulness, but let him know you really would rather be with him.

- *Tell them what you need.* If you can't continue having Christmas dinner at your house, let your family know you have to suspend that tradition for a while. If you can't stand being alone, arrange something with your family or friends for the times you know it's going to be too quiet. Ask for their patience during this temporary adjustment time.

- *Get them to read the last chapter of this book.* That chapter is specifically for them. I can say things to them that you can't.

REACH OUT AND GROUP SOMEONE

Support groups abound these days. But a key ingredient to your own growth and making it through the uglies during menopause is to get some other women around you. Perhaps you're in a situation without many close friends, or maybe you're at a loss about how to build warm relationships. I suggest you read *Friendship: Skills for Having a Friend, Being a Friend*.[2]

If you don't already have a support group, let me give you some tips on how to start one.
1. Decide who should be included.
2. Invite them for a meeting.
3. Discuss important areas of agreement:
    a. When to start
    b. Length of each meeting
    c. Where to meet
    d. Topics/materials
    e. Format of each meeting
    f. Refreshments
    g. How many weeks/months to meet
4. Make your first meeting a positive one.
    a. Go over the items you agreed upon.
    b. Keep to your format, but be flexible for needs.
    c. Announce plans for the next meeting.
5. Make your last meeting a mini-celebration.

To give you an example, I'll tell you about my Menopause Support Group. (I call it my MSG for short!)

Several years ago my friend, Anne, told me that some of her friends were praying I'd have a rough time during menopause so I'd write a book to help them! (My husband says, "Thanks a lot!") At the time, I chuckled and tucked the idea away in my brain. As the years rolled by, I indeed had menopausal difficulties and met many other women who did too. I decided that it would help me personally to have a support group.

As I considered who should be in the group, guess who was first on my list? Anne, of course. And then I thought of one of her friends who had been "praying" for me! Carol was next on the list. Right after her was Marilyn, one of our assistants at Mid-Life Dimensions. By that time, I knew I needed to watch the compatibility of the group. (Some day I'd like to have a large group open to many women, but for now I needed to keep it small.) I invited one other woman, Mary, who is Anne's sister and a professional woman who works near our office.

As I telephoned each one, they surprised me by being excited to be invited. I had thought they'd look at it as doing *me* a favor, but they each were glad to be included. We decided that the best time to meet was late in the afternoon on a day when Marilyn was at work in our office. Two of the group would be finished with their school-related work at 3:30 P.M., and the three of us would take off work in order to meet. We agreed to meet every two weeks, with adjustments as necessary. Some times we have gone a month or more between meetings.

We meet for an hour and a half in my living room. To keep the time focused on our purpose, we agreed to serve only beverages. We start with a short devotional thought and then we share menopause information and encourage each

other. We often close by praying for the specific needs that
each woman has shared during our time together. Because I
have been working on this book, my MSG friends have also
helped me with this project.

We haven't decided on a "last meeting" yet. None of us is
ready to forego the encouragement we receive from each
other.

NURTURING YOU

Part of your successful transition into this new time of
life is your responsibility to be good to yourself. This doesn't
mean you are to be self-centered toward and independent
from others, but it does mean that you provide little times of
restoration for yourself.

Women in my study who shared what was helpful to
them during menopause often mentioned that they did
special things for themselves, such as set aside a time to
read, take a special bubble bath, shop, walk in the woods, or
arrange some other little treat for themselves. Many mentioned taking time to rebuild a friendship.

You see, you can be Spartan and deny yourself little
delights, saying, "Well, that's not going to take away my
troubles anyway, so I'll just grit my teeth and carry on." Or
you can realize that by taking a few moments for refreshment,
you'll get a new grip for carrying on a little longer. When you
feel fresh, you like yourself better, and you're more ready to
connect with your world again.

Anne Morrow Lindbergh reminds us that a woman
becomes whole by becoming a "world to oneself," not to be

separate from her husband or other loved ones but to become a "world to oneself for another's sake."[3] What she means is that a woman needs to be at home with herself, and then she will be more effective in others' lives. Or, as my friend Betty Coble says in her "Woman—Aware and Choosing" workshops, "You cannot give what you do not have."[4]

If you are depleted in emotional strength, you will be of little good to yourself or anyone else. You need your inner world to be filled and at peace before your outer world can be satisfying.

SMILING AT THE FUTURE

Now I want to talk to you again as if we were face-to-face. Together we've agonized over the menopausal symptoms, feelings, and situations, and we've looked at some of the helps. I've tried to be honest, with a mixture of how awful menopause can be and how full of hope we can be for the future.

I would be negligent to give you all these pages and chapters of information and not tell you that I believe the greatest strength you can have for a successful passage through menopause is to have a personal relationship with God through Jesus Christ. Nearly every one of the 436 women who participated in my research said that knowing the Lord was very important to them.

These women were straightforward about their problems and complaints. And when asked what *helped*, along with other suggestions, they said *their spiritual life*. The majority said that it was the *most important help*. And I believe them.

You may have that same relationship or you may think that it's not for you. You may have a faith in God, but you don't acknowledge Christ as a part of your faith. Whatever your position, I'm just going to tell you that I've found the words in Proverbs 31:25, 30 to be true:

> She is a woman of strength and dignity, and has no fear of old age.

> Charm can be deceptive and beauty doesn't last, but a woman who fears and reverences God shall be greatly praised.
> (The Living Bible)

The New International Version of the Bible translates "no fear of old age" as "she can laugh at the days to come."

As we menopausal women face a multitude of changes in our lives and see how quickly youth and beauty have faded, we can actually smile at the future when we know *Who* holds it in the palm of his hand.

Another section of Scripture that I've claimed many times when things looked desperate is Isaiah 43:1-3a:

> But now the Lord who created you, O Israel, says, "Don't be afraid, for I have ransomed you; I have called you by name; you are mine. When you go through deep waters and great trouble, I will be with you. When you go through rivers of difficulty, you will not drown! When you walk through the fire of oppression, you will not be burned up—the flames will not consume you. "For I am the Lord your God, your Savior, the Holy One of Israel. . . .
> (The Living Bible)

Feel like you're drowning? Burning up? (Could those be hot flashes? I'm just teasing!) During menopause we often feel emotionally swamped, oppressed, and about to be consumed. But we have the promise that "God our Savior" is with us. His presence will carry us through the toughest times. His wisdom will point us to practical help. He is *for* us and *with* us.

We each are at different places in our spiritual journey. Some of us are just getting started; others have walked a long time with God; still others have wandered off the road for a time; and some are considering whether to even begin the journey. Those who've started the journey and have experienced the comforting, powerful presence of "God our Savior" would encourage everyone else to join them on the path.

If you'd like to know how to get started in this friendship relationship with God, here are some easy steps:

1. See your need of a Savior. (See Romans 3:23 and 6:23.)
2. Recognize that Christ paid the sacrifice for your sins, failures, shortcomings, weaknesses. (John 3:16; 1 Peter 1:19.)
3. Specifically ask Christ to forgive you. (Romans 10:13.)
4. Take possession of the new life he has given you. (2 Corinthians 5:17; Romans 5:1-2.)

I would urge you to read the Bible and pray each day. Reading the Gospel of John is a good place to start if you are unfamiliar with Scripture. Tell someone else about your new commitment to a relationship with God. And find a Bible-

believing group of people for fellowship and spiritual
strength for your new journey.

THE ADVENTURE AHEAD

We started this chapter as if we were out to run a race.
We used words like *action, on your mark, get set, know, grow,* and
other phrases that stimulate vigor and zest. Now we end by
talking of a "journey." You may see yourself at a starting line,
ready to sprint toward some goal that means victory. Or you
may picture yourself on a leisurely walk in some pleasant
spot with green grass, trees, flowers, and sparkling water.

Whatever you envision for yourself, I trust that you
possess a touch of adventure for the unexplored life ahead.
Yes, you've had to say good-bye to some dear parts of your
past, but now you can fit into the new scene that you will
help create. I hope you are now better able to "smile at the
future."

I'd like to tell you about a woman who smiles at the
future—and the present: my husband's Aunt Elsie. I have
admired her for over 37 years. Although we have been
separated by one to two thousand miles during that time, we
have seen each other periodically and keep in touch by mail
and by phone.

She recently had her 84th birthday, so that means she
was 47 when I first met her. She may have been experiencing
early menopausal symptoms, but I was unaware of them.
What I did notice about her was a warmth and graciousness
that have never diminished in all these years. She is the kind
of woman I want to be when I am her age.

She has gone through some tough problems in life, but she's a winner. She's made it into her eighties with a loving, vibrant, magnetic attitude. Life's difficulties have never been the focus of her attention. Instead, she concentrates on others, the good in the world around her, and her Creator and Savior. All who know her cherish her impact on their lives.

Since I want to be a woman like Aunt Elsie, I have studied the qualities that make her so attractive. One is that she cares for people. When you are with her, you feel as if you are the most important person in the world. She always focuses on you and your interests, not on herself. I am sure she has an extra large heart because of all the love it holds for others.

Also, Aunt Elsie believes the best about people. She tries to understand where each person is coming from and to imagine what it would be like to walk in that one's shoes. She is one older person who doesn't think "the younger generation is going to the dogs."

As much as anyone can, she keeps abreast of the latest happenings in our world. She doesn't shake her head about how fast everything is changing, but she wants to learn and grow. Consequently, it's fun to be with Aunt Elsie. She's fresh—interested and interesting.

Her husband, Art, was a pastor, and she was the kind of pastor's wife you'd want in your church. She didn't simply live out a role, however; she was a person in her own right. She received a degree in Christian Education when most women didn't even go to college, and she used her leadership abilities in many ways through the years.

Aunt Elsie and Uncle Art raised two sons who are outstanding in their Christian lives. One is a chemist, the other a pastor. They each have families who have had normal ups and downs—sicknesses, serious accidents, career and schooling detours—but they are families anyone would be proud to have. Aunt Elsie is not only a grandmother, but Aunt Elsie is also a caring great grandmother now.

Some years ago she stood alongside Uncle Art as he battled Parkinson's disease and severe arthritis. He eventually had to retire from active ministry. When he also became a cancer victim, Aunt Elsie nursed him at home for many long months before his death.

After Uncle Art died, their church asked her to be on the staff. She was already past "retirement age," but that didn't stop her from actively and lovingly working many hours a week, visiting the sick and needy, teaching classes, and performing other duties.

One time, when we were going to be passing through her city, we wrote to tell her we'd like to visit. Unknown to us, she was hospitalized with severe burns from a pressure-cooker accident. When we arrived at her son's home, there she was! She had wangled permission to leave the hospital for a few hours to be with us.

She briefly told us about her accident and then spent the afternoon concentrating on us, our ministry, and our three daughters. In fact, our girls sat on the floor by Aunt Elsie's chair for a couple of hours, asking her to tell them about herself as a young girl. They wanted to know all they could about life "back then," our family's spiritual heritage, and what she thought were important lessons for them to know for their lives. She is the kind of woman from whom teenagers wanted to learn!

In her late seventies, she decided to make plans for her future needs. She carefully researched retirement centers, personally visited some, and chose the one she felt had the best arrangement for her. She sold her small home and, with the help of her sons, moved to the center. She lives very independently in a comfortable duplex. The facility, which has several hundred residents, also has provisions for other levels of care should her health require it.

At the center Aunt Elsie started making friends with everyone around her. She was elected president of the large missionary organization, took charge of arrangements for the Sunday evening vespers, and became a Helping Friend to those who are confined to beds in the nursing care section. She reads, writes letters, and runs errands for her assigned patients. Oh, yes, she also teaches the young married couples' class at her church in a nearby town. (Remember, she's 84 years old!)

Shortly after Aunt Elsie arrived at the center, her son called to tell her he would like to visit on a certain day. She, however, was going to be so busy with her many responsibilities, she asked if he could come another day. "Imagine," he wrote to us, "my mother in a retirement center is so busy that I have to *schedule* my visits with her!"

We also scheduled a time to see her at the center. As she showed us around all the facilities, everyone called out enthusiastic greetings to her. We could tell that she was much loved and very involved with the many residents and staff at the center.

While we were there, she learned that my husband liked

baked custard. So when we had finished our tour, she went to her kitchen and whipped up a large recipe of custard for us to enjoy before we went to bed.

A couple of years later she visited us at our California home (after making adequate arrangements to be absent from her commitments at the center!). She insisted that we keep on with our work while she took care of the kitchen. During the days she was with us, she not only cooked and did dishes, she made two different batches of bread, did light office work, taught me some handcrafts, and met our friends.

Aunt Elsie is a woman you love to love! However, her qualities are not unattainable for the rest of us. She wasn't born with a silver spoon in her mouth. She has made important choices along the way that are keys to her happiness now, but life hasn't always been perfect for her. She has had her share of hurts, illnesses, death, and loneliness.

Her attitudes make the difference. Very early in her life she made a commitment to a personal relationship with Christ. Along the way, too, she learned to focus on others and developed the habit of positive thinking.

Please don't think, "Well, it's too late for me. I'm not like that."

I've learned that it's never too late to change. I've often been challenged about something I need to correct or redirect in my life, and I've found that "Old dogs *can* learn new tricks," especially when the tricks mean more successful living for myself and for others around me.

Now that I am entering a new era of life, I intend to do all I can to "smile at the future." Please, will you smile with me? Laugh out loud, if you'd like!

15

For Husbands and Children Only: Understanding "Meno Mama"

"Quit talking and get that salad put together!" I barked. My voice just hung in the air. None of my three almost-grown daughters said a word. But I was sure they were giving each other knowing glances. I was embarrassed. I hadn't meant to be cross. But I couldn't think of a good way to apologize and correct the matter.

Then I started to sniffle. I wanted to burst out crying, but this was no time to get carried away. Our friends would arrive for dinner any minute, and we still had much to do. Tense about having the meal ready on time, now I was feeling so scrambled inside, I was ready to fall apart right where I stood in the kitchen.

Sensing my predicament, one of the girls teasingly, but

lovingly, said, "Oh, Mom, you're just acting like a 'Meno Mama!'" And we all laughed.

The nickname stuck. We have used it many times over the years, and always with humor and affection. Jim and our daughters have found it to be a gentle way to warn me when I'm starting to unravel. And, to get out of awkward moments, I've called *myself* "Meno Mama."

So what about the Meno Mama at your house? Has she gone off her rocker? Are you wondering what's happened? She used to be strong and calm, the one you counted on. She always put you and the rest of the family first, before herself. She could get so much done in a day—her own jobs around the house, yours if you forgot, her work-for-pay job, extra things for other people—and she had time left over to listen to you if you ever felt like talking.

Oh, of course, she had her faults, but now—now, she's unbelievable! She falls apart, thinks only of herself, and is crabbing at you all the time. When she isn't angry, she's crying. What's going on? You know it might be time for menopause, but why all this fuss? Can't she just get her act together? After all, you have more important things to do than tip-toe around her delicate feelings.

WHAT'S GOING ON

The first 11 chapters of this book explain what's going on in your wife or mother's body, but in case you don't have time to read all that, we'll give you the information in a nutshell here. It may help you to know that, in addition to researching the latest literature and consulting with several medical experts, I have done a study of 436 menopausal women across the nation. (Look at the back of this book for a copy of the questionnaire they completed.) Also, since 1977 my husband and I have been intensely involved in helping men and women in mid-life[1]; in the course of that ministry, many menopausal women have shared their stories with us. In addition, my own personal experience validates what the experts and other women say.

My main objective in this section is to help you, the husbands and children of menopausal women, understand what's going on and how you can help. After all, it would be great if all of you could get through this time with your sanity—and your relationship with your wife or mother—intact.

The important fact for you to know is that she needs you. Her whole world may be upside down, but you can help. Her hormones are unbalanced, but something can be done about it. Other physical and emotional parts of her are out of kilter, but you can encourage her to get the help she needs.

The Big Switch

Menopause is the time when a woman's reproductive system not only shuts down but goes into reverse to a state similar to puberty. Sometime around her late forties or early fifties (the average age is 51.5), a woman's ovaries cease functioning and her menstrual periods stop. She can no longer become pregnant. Sounds simple, doesn't it? But it's not.

The glands, hormones, and reproductive organs all must

work together in the shutting-down process, and they usually don't do so harmoniously or consistently. Even when they do, it's a big change for the body after 35 to 40 years of menstrual activity.

You might compare the whole procedure to a large, complex factory, changing from making cars to building airplanes. The factory doesn't stop making cars one day and then suddenly and smoothly make airplanes the next. A whole revamping is needed, and then there may be many hitches before the factory is smoothly making the new machines.

For a woman, the transition is rarely smooth either. If her ovaries are surgically removed, everything stops at once— she's thrown into an instant menopause. As you might expect, her body doesn't suddenly and smoothly take up the new way of living. With a natural menopause, her system doesn't efficiently begin life anew either.

The Way She Was

For the 500 or so times your wife or mother has had her period in the last approximately four decades, here is very briefly what has happened. For those of you who don't need a Biology 101 refresher course, skip to the next section.

A woman's brain, by way of a hormone, signals an ovary to cause an egg to mature and to produce the hormone estrogen. Still another hormone released by the brain causes the ovary to release the egg. This process takes two weeks. The egg then travels down the fallopian tube to the uterus.

If a male sperm is present to fertilize the egg, the egg

attaches to the uterine lining, and a baby begins to grow. (The uterine lining has been prepared by estrogen and another hormone, progesterone.) If the egg is not fertilized, it is released, along with the unused uterine lining, through the vagina. Your wife or mother has her "period."

After it released the egg, the ovary began to produce progesterone, which caused the uterine lining to stop multiplying and begin maturing for a baby. As both the progesterone and estrogen levels drop, a signal is sent to the brain that the system needs to kick in again. The brain again alerts an ovary to cause an egg to mature, and so it goes, month after month, year after year, except for pregnancy or unusual trauma.

Even this simplified description gives you a sense of how complicated a women's reproductive system is, how many hormones control it, and how many places things can get out of alignment. It's understandable that things seem upside down in your wife or mother now that the routine is starting to break down.

Menopause

My husband, Jim, wonders why it isn't called "women-o-pause." And I wonder why it's called "pause" when it's never going to start up again.

Once the menopause has occurred, the reproductive system will never function again. This is because the number of eggs in each woman's ovaries declines through the years until there are no more. Thus, the hormone released by the brain has no eggs to bring to maturity, estrogen and progesterone levels drop, ovulation does not occur, the uterine lining does not build up each month, and menstruation stops.

HOT FLASHES AND OTHER CRAZINESS

As estrogen and progesterone decline, many other body functions and systems, in addition to the reproductive system, are affected. Hot flashes are often one of the earliest—and most well-known—symptoms of menopause.

These happen because the system that regulates blood vessel movement is receiving unreliable cues. Normally, the nerves that control blood vessel movement receive signals from our body temperature. If we're cold, the vessels contract and draw blood deep inside our body to conserve heat. If we're warm, the vessels expand, allowing the blood to be near the skin surface to let the heat out. A woman's hormones help transmit messages to the nerves. When her hormones become erratic, the signals to the nerves do too. Dizziness, heart palpitations, tingling skin, and jumpiness may also occur from these faulty signals.

You thought she was just being cantankerous when she flinched and complained about your driving. She was sure you hadn't seen that car pulling out from that side street! Be patient with her. Her reactions to stimuli are way off now. She's not just being emotional; this is a physical, biological symptom.

Eventually, you will notice other physical changes. Her skin and tissues change. It's not simply aging: it's from a lack of estrogen. Membranes become thin and dry. Her face and hands become wrinkled. She is more prone to vaginal and urinary burning, irritation, and infection. She may leak urine when she sneezes, coughs, or jumps. Vaginal lubrication may drastically decrease and tissues become thin and fragile so that intercourse becomes painful. In time, the shape and size of the vagina will become smaller so that intercourse may become impossible.

Don't panic! Intervention and prevention are available, as you'll see in a few pages.

While your Meno Mama is battling deteriorating tissues, she may also be fighting pain in her muscles and joints. She may not be sleeping well, and she may be tired much of the time.

When I was in the throes of the worst menopausal symptoms, I would awaken in the middle of the night, feeling like a shot of adrenalin had burst through me. I would be as alert as if I'd just found a hundred dollar bill on the street.

I'd tell myself to relax and go back to sleep, because I needed my energy for the full day coming up. Counting sheep would turn into counting things I had to remember to do once I got up. I'd have to keep rehearsing them, so I didn't forget any. Of course, I couldn't drop off to sleep then.

I finally resorted to keeping a pencil and paper on the night stand, so I could reach over in the dark and jot down my notes. Jim compared me to a hamster—up scratching around all night!

IN YEARS TO COME....

These immediate symptoms, which can last from a few months to many years, are bad enough, but your wife and mother's future health is also at stake. With the decline of estrogen, she is much more apt to become a victim of osteoporosis, the deteriorating bone disease that affects at least one-third—and maybe as many as one-half—of all postmenopausal women. She may eventually fracture her vertebrae, hip, pelvis, ankle, or arm. Even if she sustains no major fracture, she will live with pain as she is losing bone mass.

Your wife's risk of heart disease also rises after menopause: she is as liable to have a heart attack as men are and more likely than men to have a stroke. And don't forget the natural aging processes, such as changing body shape, wrinkles, gray hair, and loss of strength and stamina. These affect both men and women, but they occur more rapidly in postmenopausal women!

ROLLER-COASTER FEELINGS

The 436 women in my survey compared their emotions to a roller coaster more than any other image. They also used the phrase "out of control" more than any other. For most women these are new experiences. Some women may have had PMS (Premenstrual Syndrome), but menopause is usually worse.

For reasons not yet clearly understood by scientists, a woman's dropping estrogen level affects her whole emotional/psychological functioning. During menopause a woman's feelings are less dependable than the weather. The fluctuations are hard on everyone around, especially her.

One moment she feels intensely angry at things that

never used to upset her; the next moment she is choking back tears. She's embarrassed to feel so overly sensitive about little issues. She is insecure, suspicious, and jealous. Anxiety sweeps over her like an unwanted blast of cold air.

CHANGING IDENTITY

As if all the physical upheavals aren't enough for your wife or mother, they usually occur at a time when her roles and relationships are undergoing drastic modifications. Her grown or nearly grown children are needing her less, so her job description is changing. She will need to adapt to life in a nest without the chicks. As the children marry and have children, she becomes a mother-in-law and a grandma, with all the positives and negatives those roles may bring.

If you, her husband, are preoccupied with work or feel less affectionate toward her, she may feel like a displaced person. Even if your relationship is happy, she will still need to restructure her identity in the light of all the changes.

About now, too, she begins a new parenting process—that of caring for her (and maybe your) aging parents. Although she may not be completely responsible for their daily needs, she realizes she has an increased obligation for their happiness and welfare. She remembers what they once did for her.

Career roles may change too. Your wife at this age, for the first time, may be free to start pursuing a profession of her own. She may want some additional education. Or she may have had a career for a long time and find it changing. She may be facing age discrimination or early retirement.

Take Elaine, for example. She had taught school before she was married and for most of the years her children were growing up. She had about 10 or 12 years to go before retirement when her husband decided to retire early. He wanted to travel, and he wanted Elaine to come along. He set up some part-time consulting jobs in other states to pay their expenses as they enjoyed their adventures.

Elaine was excited to go, but she found herself explaining to everyone, "I took an *early* retirement," so they would know she wasn't really old enough to retire. She found it hard being introduced as a "former teacher."

When her husband decided, after several months and thousands of miles, not to travel so much and to open a consulting office at home, Elaine suffered an identity crisis. She had spent nearly 30 years going to work every day. It was often a grind, but she was needed and the fulfillment outweighed the strain. Now, it seemed only her house needed her. She could enjoy doing housework only so many hours a day and then she needed other stimulation.

Elaine spent several months in a miserable state of depression and questioning. She had never felt so useless. She enjoyed the freedom from demands of a full-time career, but trying to identify her new place in life was terribly painful. She was even uncertain how to go about finding what steps to take next.

Finally Elaine took a part-time job. It was very rewarding. She also saw a doctor and started on estrogen replacement. About the same time, her daughter and husband moved near them, and in a few months her first grandchild was born. She now had the joy of caring for the baby at least once a week while her daughter had a day out.

Elaine feels that her life has finally come together again, but it took more than three years. When she evaluates what helped her, she credits estrogen, the new baby, and her job. "Oh, yes," she adds, "And my husband was very patient during all my upheaval."

WHAT YOU CAN DO TO HELP

One of the most helpful things you can do for your wife or your mother as she goes through the symptoms of menopause is to *assure her that she is normal*. Don't tell her that she is just being weak or wanting sympathy. Avoid making her feel guilty. One of the worst things you can do is to say—or imply—that she has a spiritual or psychological deficiency.

One of the women in my study wrote, "The most difficult part of menopause was that my husband did not understand and would not believe me when I tried to explain what was happening to me. He believed it was a spiritual problem. His attitude has done great emotional damage to me, which will take years to overcome."

This same woman wrote in the space provided for what was "most helpful" during menopause: "My children were very supportive even though it was a strain on them."

Another menopausal woman I'll call Fran was the wife of a doctor. Some of their children were grown and gone, but a son and daughter were still at home. Both were rebelling against all of their family's values, but Fran was especially grieved about her daughter Cindy's apparent sexual activity.

Fran tried every method to talk to her, befriend her, and help her out of her destructive lifestyle, but the girl acted as if she despised her mother's love and concern. Cindy knew her mother was going through menopause. But she had no regard for her mother's needs, and she absolutely refused to accept any tenderness from Fran. This pain with Cindy compounded the distress of Fran's severe menopause symptoms.

Fran's husband was consumed with his medical practice and golf games. Fran tried to enlist his help with their daughter and son, but he was preoccupied. She also wanted his care for her menopause symptoms, but he either ignored her or got angry when she couldn't keep herself under control. In addition, he didn't want her to go for help from any other doctor at the clinic. He said he didn't want to be embarrassed.

Then Fran learned that her husband was emotionally involved with one of the nurses at the clinic. The next week they found Fran hanging by a rope from a rafter in the family's three-car garage.

As husband or children, you have the opportunity for helping "make or break" the menopausal woman in your life. It isn't all up to you, of course, but you are an important key to her successfully making it through these rough years.

Probably, before you can assure Meno Mama that she is normal, however, you have to be convinced yourself. I would urge you to read this entire book or one of the books listed in the *Bibliography* so that you understand more about menopause. Once you realize the gigantic physical changes that are taking place, you will know your wife or mother is normal—for a menopausal woman. The good news is that she will eventually pass through this stage. And you can help make the passage smoother.

YOUR QUIET MERCY

Patience may need to be your prime virtue during this time. Your wife or mother probably seems so unreasonable that you just want to tell her off or run off. Instead, try to take a deep breath, murmur a prayer for wisdom, and gently stand alongside her. She needs your non-condemning friendship.

Remember the times you too have needed unconditional love. She probably helped provide it. She'll some day again be her rational, caring self. Once she gets through menopause, she might be even better than before. If the important people around her have helped her during her crisis, she may have grown and learned so much that her good qualities will just naturally overflow.

You may wonder what you're supposed to do about *honesty* in your relationship with Meno Mama. Is she just supposed to get away with murder? Are you simply to let her carry on with her distorted perceptions, hateful remarks, and selfish actions?

Mercy and tolerance *are* important attributes for you in this situation. At times you will need to help her see that she's wrong, but do so gently, remembering that you might need similar help someday.[2] How would you want to be treated?

Choose the best timing for talking to her. Don't confront

her in the middle of a crisis. Wait until she's calmer and more objective.

Positive actions and attitudes will be more effective than talk. I see myself more clearly and can better evaluate where I need to change when Jim and my daughters combine love, patience, and confidence in me with their words.

You don't have to be a doormat during this time, but do be wise about *how, when,* and *how much* you say. Your cheerful, tender respect will go a long way in helping the menopausal woman in your life. Think of it as turning the other cheek or walking the second mile.[3] You'll survive, even if you have to go ten or twenty extra miles! And your relationship will get better.

YOUR MEDICAL COUNSEL

One of the best ways to help your menopausal wife or mother is to urge her to *see a good doctor* who will work with her in managing her menopausal symptoms. If the first doctor isn't a help, encourage her to find another. You cannot believe how many women (at least 75 percent in my survey) have trouble finding a competent doctor who adequately cares for their needs during menopause. As a family member, you can encourage her not to give up in her search for the help she needs.

If her doctor feels she is a candidate for *hormone replacement therapy,* stand behind the idea 100 percent. I know of many husbands and children who, as one man said, "want to sing an ode to estrogen" for the great changes it brings about in the menopausal woman at their house. As another man said, "I feel as if I have my wife back again."

My friend Connie tells of her teenage daughter, Jill, being able to sense when it was time for Connie to have another estrogen injection. Jill could tell it before her mother could. (That's usually the case!)

Without realizing it, Connie's voice would begin to sound tired and whiny, she'd become cross and irritable, and she wouldn't feel like tackling her housework. Jill would say, "Mom, isn't it about time for another shot of estrogen?"

Jill's reminder would cause Connie to check the calendar and see that it was indeed time for another injection. After she had the shot, she would then bounce back to being herself for a few more weeks.

If you are wondering about whether estrogen is necessary or safe, I would suggest you read Chapter 6 of this book or some of the books listed in the *Bibliography*.

The benefits of estrogen replacement therapy (ERT) or hormone replacement therapy (HRT—estrogen plus progesterone) include the following:

- Emotional and psychological stabilization
- Elimination of hot flashes
- Reduction of tissue deterioration (fewer wrinkles, healthier urinary and vaginal areas)
- Maintenance of sexual libido and possibility for intercourse
- Prevention or reduction in risk of bone deterioration (osteoporosis)
- Prevention or reduction in risk of heart attack and stroke (cardiovascular disease)

Urge your menopausal woman to get the health care she needs for the rest of her body too, including *annual breast examinations and mammograms*. One of every ten women will get breast cancer, but the chances of recovery are very high when detected early.

Encourage her to *eat correctly and exercise*. Don't nag, but affirm her when she recognizes the need to watch her weight. Criticism and underhanded digs will have a negative effect. Instead, join her in eating plans to help her lose weight even if you don't need to lose. Go walking with her several times a week. Buy her a nice running outfit. Jim and my daughters have done these things for me throughout these last years, and it has been easier for me to be disciplined.

As a gift to your wife or mother, *watch your own health*. Get your physical checkups, watch your food intake, exercise regularly—and, if you smoke or drink, stop. (Men who use alcohol or nicotine get osteoporosis too.) If you take care of your health, your menopausal woman can stop worrying about you, and you will inspire her to care for herself.

YOUR SEXUAL HELP

For sons or daughters: Encourage your mother to get the medical help she needs so that her sexual life with her husband stays—or becomes—vital. Diplomatically urge him to do his part too by being romantic with her and getting medical help if he needs it.

Husbands: Here are some tips for you:

• *Help your wife feel sexy.* What you say and how you treat her changing body is very important in how she will respond to you. Remember that you also are aging. Let her know you find her attractive. If certain clothes or actions stimulate you, tell her.

• *Make yourself desirable too.* Many women complain that it's hard to enjoy sexual intimacy with husbands who are overweight, smelly, or inattentive except when they want sex.

• *Be gentle.* Because her vaginal tissues may be dry and tender, don't be rough with her. A little patience at the beginning of intercourse will make the experience much more pleasant for her and make her more willing the next time.

She may not let you know how painful intercourse is, or she may disrupt the entire atmosphere by being angry with you for being thoughtless. Talk to her about it. Ask if you are hurting her.

Encourage her to use one of the available preparations to help with lubrication. If her doctor says it's safe, urge her to use estrogen replacement therapy by pill or skin patch to prevent deterioration of her vaginal structure and to lessen the risk of urinary and vaginal infections.

• *Be loving at times other than when you want to have sex.* I'm sure you're aware of women's age-old grievance that their husbands only show affection when they want to get them into bed. Your attitudes, words, and actions all day long contribute to successful lovemaking.

● *Be loyal to your wife.* Whatever kind of marriage ceremony you had, you promised to be faithful. Nothing erodes a sexual relationship with your wife faster than adultery or the suspicion of it—or if you act as if that's what you're looking for by the attentions you give other women.

If your honor isn't sufficient to keep your marriage bed sacred, at least be concerned about the horrendous potential of AIDS and other sexually transmitted diseases. If you are being tempted to have an affair, be smart enough to get counseling to make your marriage strong and satisfying.

● *Let your wife know about your sexual changes.* Unless you are many years younger than she, you too are probably very different during intercourse than you were years ago. You may be slower in obtaining and maintaining an erection or in reaching ejaculation. You may not have the energy for sex at bedtime, but you may be ready after a night's rest.

Talk about these matters with your wife. You may find great satisfaction in just holding and caressing each other without the affection always culminating in intercourse. Together the two of you can discover the joys of a sexual relationship that may be better than in your early years.

YOUR TANGIBLE ASSISTANCE

For sons, daughters, and husbands: Some other ways to help your wife or mother are in actual *physical labor.* Many women are worn out by the time of menopause. For decades, they have been doing much of the housework, working part-time or full-time, and carrying most of the responsibility for the little and big things that make family relationships flourish.

This is a good time for you to take on more of the responsibilities that traditionally have been hers. Don't wait to be asked. Cook, clean, do the laundry, and shop for groceries. Change the sheets. Write the Christmas thank-you notes. Telephone Grandma to see how she is. Clean up after yourself. Quit expecting to be waited on; wait on her some of the time.

As you help around the house more, you may lower your expectations about how things need to be done. Perhaps you'll be happy with simpler meals. You'll understand if the shirts need to be sent out to be ironed. You might even insist on hiring someone to clean house every week or two.

Several years ago Jim told me I had cleaned enough toilets for a lifetime. I didn't need to do any more to build my character! He urged me to get someone to clean our house regularly so that I would be free to do "more important" things.

He has always helped around the house, but he's more fully shared the nitty-gritty household tasks in recent years. I don't know how I would have managed to care for everything else without his help during my menopausal years when my physical strength and motivation were reduced.

YOUR STRONG ENCOURAGEMENT

Besides caring physically for your wife or mother, you can be her biggest *emotional booster*. She often may lack the inner strength or physical energy for activities that used to come easily. Assure her that it's all right to let things slide for a season.

Urge her to rest when she's tired. Encourage her to do things that will nourish and replenish her spirit. For some women, refreshment comes from shopping; for others, it's the opportunity to read, take a brisk walk, refinish a chair, or be with friends. Provide opportunies for her to do what *she* finds relaxing.

She'll need continual times of restoration. One time doesn't do it. She'll feel better for a while, but then her emotional sponge will start drying out again. She may need "permission" from you to keep doing the things that will rebuild her.

Be sensitive to what she needs. Sometimes she will want time with you; sometimes she will need to be alone. At times she will want to be with a big crowd of people; other times she will want to withdraw. Don't be dismayed if one of these extremes lasts for months. She'll eventually get back into balance.

Encourage her to follow her dreams. When she starts sorting through the confusion of her changing body and new roles, help her to set and get excited about new goals. Tell her what you see as her strengths and abilities. Point out her opportunities.

Do your part to make it possible for her to go back to school, start a new career, develop a neglected hobby, spend more time with the grandchildren, or whatever she senses would bring fulfillment. She needs to be moving into God's plan for her in this new era of life.

YOUR PART IN HER SELF-CONCEPT

I think most husbands and children don't realize how crucial their input is to the menopausal woman's self-image. Yes, I know we menopausal women are supposed to be all grown up and mature about such things. But the longer I live and the more women I talk to, the more I see that our identity and self-esteem are in a constant state of change all through life.

During menopause and the years following, self-esteem can shrivel like a mushroom in the sun. Some women I've known were originally self-confident, but when estrogen began to depart, so did their self-esteem. Imagine what happens to women who had a *poor* self-image before menopause!

A woman's low self-esteem is exaggerated by her hormonal imbalance, and it also is affected by the drastic changes in her body, role in life, and important relationships. Some might argue that the lack of estrogen has nothing to do with her view of herself, but I've known the same woman's self-image to improve greatly when estrogen replacement starts. I'm one of them. And many women in my survey agreed.

Most women will be glad when they've reached the place where their security and value come from their knowledge of God's view of them, rather than from balanced hormones or harmonious circumstances and relationships. But that's an ideal state not usually experienced by a woman during the instability of menopause.

Until then, what can you do? First of all realize how important you are to your wife or mother as a *builder* of her self-esteem. Following are some very practical building blocks:

- *Give her at least one genuine compliment a day*. You can start by praising her for what she does or how she looks, but go beyond that to qualities of her character. Personality traits are more lasting than performance or appearance. Give her something that will endure if she can no longer "do" or "look so good." After you've practiced one compliment a day, begin increasing the number.

- *Hug her*. We've been learning in recent decades how important physical touch is for emotional health. Meno Mama is in *great need* of some warm and spontaneous daily hugs. Other affection is important too. Husbands, use those lovemaking tips we gave earlier.

- *Keep—or develop—positive attitudes toward her*. If she has just said something off the wall or she's having an appalling hot flash in public, don't roll your eyes and act as if she's crazy. Treat her with dignity, not disgust. She may be having troubles but she's not stupid. Your manner toward her can either enhance her view of herself or totally destroy it.

- *Give her an accurate, positive reflection of her strengths and capabilities*. She probably can only see her weaknesses. What you think about her can be very constructive in building her self-esteem and helping her set new goals. Let her know the good qualities and abilities you see in her.

- *Give her the assurance that you believe in her.* Of course, she's not perfect. Neither are you. But if you let her know you're sure she's going to come through this time a better woman, she'll probably fulfill your prophecy.

You have a big assignment, but not an impossible one. You know that God has made your menopausal wife or mother to be a special woman. Be sure to tell her that often. Encourage her with these words:

I am sure that God who began the good work within you will keep right on helping you grow in his grace until his task within you is finally finished on that day when Jesus Christ returns. (Philippians 1:6, The Living Bible)

About the Author

SALLY CHRISTON CONWAY is co-founder and vice-president of Mid-Life Dimensions (Christian Living Resources, Inc.), a non-profit speaking, counseling, and writing ministry designed to help people in mid-life.

She is author of *Your Husband's Mid-Life Crisis* and coauthor of *Women in Mid-Life Crisis*, *Your Marriage Can Survive Mid-Life Crisis*, and *What God Gives When Life Takes*. She has also contributed to magazines and other books.

Conway earned her B.S. in Education in 1974 and her M.S. in Human Development and Family Ecology in 1986, both from the University of Illinois in Urbana.

She and her husband, Jim, have three married daughters and several grandchildren.

Sally Conway may be contacted at the following address for speaking engagements:

Mid-Life Dimensions
P.O. Box 3790
Fullerton, CA 92634

Notes

CHAPTER 1: YOU ARE HERE

[1]My husband, Jim Conway, and I founded Mid-Life Dimensions (Christian Living Resources, Inc.), a speaking, counseling, and writing ministry, to help people in mid-life. Books we have previously authored are listed in the Bibliography.

[2]Lila Nachtigall and Joan Rattner Heilman, Estrogen: The Facts Can Change Your Life (Los Angeles: The Body Press, 1986) 7; Nissa Simon, "An Update on Estrogen-Replacement Therapy," Working Woman 14 (May 1989) 148; Cory SerVaas, "More About Estrogen Skin Patches" Saturday Evening Post 259 (Jan./Feb. 1987), 52.

[3]Chris Raymond, "Good News About Menopause: Family Troubles, Not the Climacteric, Cause Midlife Blues," American Health: Fitness of Body and Mind 7 (November 1988), 52.

[4]Pamela King, "The Meno-pause That Refreshes," Psychology Today 22 (December 1988), 11.

[5]Joanna Torrey, "Fatal Reactions: Am I Blue" (Depression in Women Over 40), Harper's Bazaar 121 (August 1988), 154.

CHAPTER 2: FIRST-TIME CHANGES FOR YOU

[1]Penny Wise Budoff, No More Hot Flashes and Other Good News (New York: Warner, 1984), 2.

[2]Ada Kahn and Linda Hughey Holt, Midlife Health (New York: Avon, 1987), 57; Nachtigall and Heilman, 192.

[3]For example, see Nachtigall and Heilman, 64.

[4]Nachtigall and Heilman, 70–71.

[5]Jim Conway, Men in Mid-Life Crisis (Elgin, Ill.: David C. Cook, 1978); Sally Conway, Your Husband's Mid-Life Crisis (Elgin, Ill.: David C. Cook, 1980).

[6]Jim and Sally Conway, Women in Mid-Life Crisis (Wheaton, Ill.: Tyndale House, 1983).

CHAPTER 3: OUR FOREMOTHERS

[1]Lila Nachtigall and Joan Rattner Heilman, Estrogen: The Facts Can Change Your Life (Los Angeles: The Body Press, 1986), 13.

[2]Nachtigall and Heilman, 13; Mary K. Beard and Lindsay Curtis, Menopause and the Years Ahead (Tucson: Fisher Books, 1988), 251.

[3]Charles D. Meigs, Woman: Her Diseases and Remedies, Letters to His Class, 3rd rev. ed. (Philadelphia: Blanchard and Lea, 1854).

[4]Catharine Beecher, Letters to the People on Health and Happiness (New York: Arno Press, 1972, originally published, New York: Harper and Row, 1855).

[5]Elizabeth Blackwell, Pioneer Work for Woman (New York: E. P. Dutton, 1914).

[6]Edward H. Clarke, Sex in Education; or A Fair Chance for Girls (Boston: James R. Osgood, 1914).

[7]Edward H. Dixon, Woman and Her Diseases from the Cradle to the Grave, 5th rev. ed. (New York, Charles H. Ring, 1847).

[8]Jane Page, The Other Awkward Age: Menopause (Berkeley: Ten Speed Press, 1977), 66.

[9]Page, 67.

[10]Page, 69.

[11]Page, 68.

[12]Page, 68.

[13]Page, 71.

[14]Margaret Mead, Male and Female (London: Victor Gollancz, 1949).

[15]Paula Weideger, Menstruation and Menopause: The Physiology and Psychology: The Myth and the Reality (New York: Delta Books, 1977).

[16]Pauline Bart, "Depression in Middle-Aged Women," *Women in Sexist Society*, ed. V. Gornick and B. K. Moran (New York, Basic Books, 1971).

[17]Nachtigall and Heilman, 14–15.

[18]Ann Mankowitz, *Change of Life: A Psychological Study of Dreams and Menopause* (Toronto: Inner City Books, 1984), 70

CHAPTER 4: YOUR WONDERFUL BODY

[1]Penny Wise Budoff, *No More Hot Flashes and Other Good News* (New York: Warner, 1984); Orene V. Schoenfeld and Beverly Bush Smith, *Change for the Better* (Old Tappan, N.J.: Fleming H. Revell, 1986).

[2]Dr. A. F. Haney, Duke University, in Mary K. Beard and Lindsay Curtis, *Menopause and the Years Ahead* (Tucson: Fisher Books, 1988), 1.

[3]*Guidelines for Perinatal Care*, 2nd ed. (American Academy of Pediatrics and American College of Obstetrics-Gynecology, 1988), 236.

[4]For example, see Sadja Greenwood, *Menopause, Naturally* (Volcano, Calif.: Volcano Press, 1989), 31; Harris H. McIlwain, Debra Fulghum Bruce, Joel C. Silverfield, and Michael C. Burnette, *Osteoporosis: Prevention, Management, Treatment* (New York: John Wiley & Sons, 1988), 27.

[5]Beard and Curtis, 10.

[6]Lila Nachtigall and Joan Rattner Heilman, *Estrogen: The Facts Can Change Your Life* (Los Angeles: The Body Press, 1986), 52.

CHAPTER 5: NOW THAT REPRODUCTION IS OVER

[1]Lila Nachtigall and Joan Rattner Heilman, *Estrogen: The Facts Can Change Your Life* (Los Angeles: The Body Press, 1986), 75.

[2]These suggestions have been gleaned from a number of sources, including my physician and Nachtigall, 109-110.

CHAPTER 6: THE ESTROGEN QUESTION

[1]Lila Nachtigall and Joan Rattner Heilman, *Estrogen: The Facts Can Change Your Life* (Los Angeles: The Body Press, 1986), 25–27, 20–22;

Penny Wise Budoff *No More Hot Flashes and Other Good News* (New York: Warner, 1984), 42–46.

[2]Nachtigall and Heilman, 26.

[3]Nachtigall and Heilman, 24.

[4]Budoff, 4.

[5]W. B. Kennel, "Metabolic Risk Factors for Coronary Heart Disease in Women: Perspective from the Framingham Study," *American Heart Journal* 114 (1987) 413–419.

[6]L. G. Raisz, "Preventing Osteoporosis by Estrogen Replacement," *Journal of Musculoskeletal Medicine* 2 (1985), 25–36; L. R. Hedlund and J. C. Gallagher, "Estrogen Therapy for Postmenopausal Osteoporosis: Current Status," *Geriatric Medicine Today* 7 (1988), 55–63; Nachtigall and Heilman, 115–17.

[7]Lila Nachtigall and Joan Rattner Heilman, *Estrogen: The Facts Can Change Your Life* (Los Angeles: The Body Press, 1986).

[8]Nachtigall and Heilman, 19, 30.

[9]Budoff, xii.

[10]Mary K. Beard and Lindsay Curtis, *Menopause and the Years Ahead* (Tucson: Fisher Books, 1988), 163, 190.

[11] Claus Christiansen, "Selection of Postmenopausal Women for Estrogen Therapy," at conference on Long-Term Effects of Estrogen Deprivation; *Postgraduate Medicine: A Special Report* (April 1989), 44, 91; Rogerio Lobo, "Summary" at conference on Long-Term Effects of Estrogen Deprivation, p. 91.

[12]Wulf H. Utian, "Renewing Our Commitment to the Remaining 85%," *Menopause Management* 2, no. 1 (Winter 1989), 2.

[13]Beard and Curtis, 169.

[14]Many sources discuss this; for example, see Nachtigall and Heilman, 36–37.

[15]For example, see Nachtigall and Heilman, 35.

[16]For example, see Nachtigall and Heilman, 35–36.

[17]For example, see Nachtigall and Heilman, 33–34, as well as Kenneth H. Cooper, *Preventing Osteoporosis* (New York: Bantam, 1989), 95.

[18]Nachtigall and Heilman, 140–41.

[19]Nachtigall and Heilman, 140.

[20]Nachtigall and Heilman, 70–71.

[21]For example, see Cooper, 97.

[22]Howard M. Fillit, "Might Estrogen Prevent Memory Loss?" Address given at a seminar, "Hormones and the Brain: The Neuroendocrinology of Aging, Alzheimer's, Stress, Depressive Illness, and Appetite Disorders," Rockefeller University Council in *Saturday Evening Post*, 258 (December 1986), 50–52, 110.

[23]Philip Sarrel and Lorna Sarrel, *Sexual Turning Points: The Seven Stages of Adult Sexuality* (New York: Macmillan & Co., 1984).

[24]Beard and Curtis, 226.

[25]Nachtigall and Heilman, 178.

[26]For example, see Nachtigall and Heiman, 187–88.

[27]Cooper, 97.

[28]James Dobson, *What Wives Wish Their Husbands Knew About Women* (Wheaton, Ill.: Tyndale House, 1975).

[29]"If you want to know what God wants you to do, ask him, and he will gladly tell you, for he is always ready to give a bountiful supply of wisdom to all who ask him" (James 1:5, Living Bible).

CHAPTER 7: HYSTERECTOMY—PRO AND CON

[1]National Center for Health Statistics, 1987, in Catherine Houck, "What Doctors Don't Tell Women about Hysterectomy," *Woman's Day* (June 16, 1987), 38.

[2]Blue Cross and Blue Shield of Greater New York, 1983, in Herbert H. Keyser, *Women Under the Knife* (Philadelphia: George F. Stickley, 1984), 41; *The New Our Bodies, Ourselves*, Boston Women's Health Book Collective, in Houck, 40.

[3]The Center for Disease Control, *Medical World News*, in Penny Wise Budoff, *No More Hot Flashes and Other Good News* (New York: Warner, 1984), 131.

[4]Houck, 38.

[5]Keyser, 41–55.

[6]Budoff, 130.

[7]Ada Kahn and Linda Hughey Holt, *Midlife Health* (New York: Avon, 1987), 64.

[8]Keyser, 41–42.

[9]Keyser, 42.

[10]Many of these questions were suggested by the material in Orene Schoenfeld and Beverly Bush Smith, *Change for the Better* (Old Tappan, N.J.: Fleming H. Revell, 1986), 135–157.

[11]Becki Conway Sanders and Jim and Sally Conway, *What God Gives When Life Takes* (Downers Grove, Ill.: InterVarsity Press, 1989).

[12]Helen Passwater, "For What Might Have Been," in Jim and Sally Conway, *Women in Mid-Life Crisis* (Wheaton, Ill.: Tyndale House, 1983), 22–23.

CHAPTER 8: THE JOY—OR PAIN—OF SEX

[1]Lila Nachtigall and Joan Rattner Heilman, *Estrogen: The Facts Can Change Your Life* (Los Angeles: The Body Press, 1986), 84.

[2]Jim and Sally Conway, *Your Marriage Can Survive Mid-Life Crisis: Ten Keys to an Intimate Marriage* (Nashville: Thomas Nelson, 1987).

[3]Conway, *Your Marriage Can Survive Mid-Life Crisis*, 232–37.

[4]Mary K. Beard and Lindsay Curtis, *Menopause and the Years Ahead* (Tucson: Fisher, 1988), 82.

[5]Nachtigall and Heilman, 92–93.

[6]Nachtigall and Heilman, 89–90.

[7]Nachtigall and Heilman, 91.

CHAPTER 9: OSTEOPOROSIS—THE SILENT THIEF

[1]Mary K. Beard and Lindsay Curtis, *Menopause and the Years Ahead* (Tucson: Fisher Books, 1988), 227.

[2]Beard and Curtis, 227.

[3]Kenneth H. Cooper, *Preventing Osteoporosis* (New York: Bantam, 1989), 7.

Orene V. Schoenfeld and Beverly Bush Smith, *Change for the Better* (Old Tappan, N.J.: Fleming H. Revell, 1986), 75.

[4]Beard and Curtis, 231.

[5]*New England Journal of Medicine* (June 26, 1986) in Cooper, 7.
[6]Lila Nachtigall and Joan Rattner Heilman, *Estrogen: The Facts Can Change Your Life* (Los Angeles: The Body Press, 1986), 117.
[7]*New England Journal of Medicine* (June 26, 1986), in Cooper, 7.
[8]Nachtigall and Heilman, 117.
[9]Compiled from Cooper, 14-25; Nachtigall and Heilman, 119-20; and Harris H. McIlwain, Debra Fulghum Bruce, Joel C. Silverfield, and Michael C. Burnette, *Osteoporosis: Prevention, Management, Treatment* (New York: John Wiley & Sons, 1988), 21.
[10]For example, see Nachtigall and Heilman, 120.
[11]Cooper, 15.
[12]Cooper, 15.
[13]For example, see Nachtigall and Heilman, 122-23.
[14]Cooper, *Preventing Osteoporosis* (New York: Bantam, 1989).
[15]McIlwain et al. *Osteoporosis: Prevention, Management, Treatment* (New York: John Wiley & Sons, 1988).

CHAPTER 10: COMBATING HEART ATTACKS AND OTHER ASSAULTS

[1]For example, see John C. Larosa, "Cardiovascular Disease in Women a Growing Concern," Prevention and Management of Cardiovascular Risk in Women: 1989 Consensus Conference on Sex Hormones in Women, *Symposia Reporter*, (Secaucus, N.J.) 13, no. 4 (October 1989), 2; American Heart Association on CNN (Cable News Network) (January 14, 1990), and in "Majority of Women Over 55 at Risk of Heart Disease," *Orange County Register* (January 15, 1990), A1; Penny Wise Budoff, *No More Hot Flashes and Other Good News* (New York: Warner, 1984), 35; and Sharon Sneed and David Sneed, *Prime Time: A Complete Health Guide for Women 35 to 65*, (Dallas: Word, 1989), 169.

[2]Trudy L. Bush, "Study of Hormone Replacement Therapy in Postmenopausal Women—the PEPI Trial—to be Launched," Prevention and Management of Cardiovascular Risk in Women: 1989 Consensus Conference on Sex Hormones in Women, *Symposia Reporter* (Secaucus, N.J.), 13, no. 4 (October 1989), 10.

[3] Bush, 10.

[4] CNN report (January 14, 1990), and *Orange County Register*, (January 15, 1990).

[5] William P. Castelli, in "How ERT Influences Cardiovascular Disease," Symposium on Heart Disease, in *Contemporary Ob/Gyn* (November 1988), 108.

[6] Sneed and Sneed, 170, a personal conversation with a physician (January 18, 1990).

[7] Leon Speroff, "Ob/Gyn's Role in Hormone Replacement Therapy and Prevention of CV Disease," Prevention and Management of Cardiovascular Risk in Women: 1989 Consensus Conference on Sex Hormones in Women, *Symposia Reporter* (Secaucus, N.J.) 13, no 4, (October 1989), 5.

[8] Speroff, 6.

[9] Journal of American Medical Association (1983) in Mary K. Beard and Lindsay Curtis, *Menopause and the Years Ahead* (Tucson: Fisher, 1988), 226.

[10] Gladys Lindberg and Judy Lindberg McFarland, *Take Charge of Your Health* (San Francisco: Harper & Row, 1982), 77; and conversation with Dr. Dwight Jordan (January 18, 1990).

[11] We also have been scared off from eating certain foods that might cause high cholesterol, but sometimes we haven't been given the total story. For example, reports about egg yolks being bad for our cholesterol level have overlooked the fact that eggs also contain lecithin and other ingredients important in *controlling* cholesterol. Some experiments to prove the danger of eggs have been conducted on animals that are vegetarians (rabbits, for instance). Because these animals would never naturally eat an egg and their bodies cannot metabolize the substances found in eggs, the results of tests on them can't be extended to humans, who are carnivorous beings. Sometimes we are being warned against foods that nature has provided and that our ancestors ate without harm. For more information, a good source to read is Lindberg and McFarland, especially 76-97.

[12] Sneed and Sneed, 173.

[13]Lila Nachtigall and Joan Rattner Heilman, *Estrogen: The Facts Can Change Your Life* (Los Angeles: The Body Press, 1986), 30.

[14]"Nurses' Health Study on Past Use of OCS and Heart Attacks," Prevention and Management of Cardiovascular Risk in Women: 1989 Consensus Conference on Sex Hormones in Women, *Symposia Reporter* (Secaucus, N.J.) 13, no. 4 (October 1989), 14; and Trudy Bush, "How ERT Influences Cardiovascular Disease," Symposium on Heart Disease in Contemporary Ob/Gyn (November 1988), 118.

[15]"Nurses' Health Study on Past OCS and Heart Attacks," 1989 Consensus Conference on Sex Hormones in Women, *Symposia Reporter*, 14.

[16]Annlia Paganini-Hill, "Estrogen Replacement Therapy and Vascular Disease: The Leisure World Study," *Postgraduate Medicine* (A Special Report on Long-Term Effects of Estrogen Deprivation) (April 1989), 49.

[17]Sources for further study are found in the notes listed above for this chapter. In addition, you may want to see the following: *The Journal of Reproductive Medicine* 30, no. 10 supplement (October 1985); Estrogen Replacement Therapy Symposium Proceedings, *International Journal of Fertility* (April 1985, supplement issue 1986; *Menopausal Update*, ed. Morris Notelovitz (Newtown, Pa.: Associates in Medical Marketing Co., Inc.), 2, no. 1; Isaac Schiff, "Is ERT Cardioprotective?" *Menopause Management* (Denville, N.J.: The Conwood Group, Inc.) 2, no. 2 (Summer 1989), 5-7; and the entire report in *Postgraduate Medicine*, 44-91.

Major studies to which references are often made in the research literature include: "*Framingham Heart Study*. The study was begun in 1948 to 'measure certain constitutional factors and certain of the conditioning factors' associated with the development of atherosclerotic and hypertensive cardiovascular diseases. The original cohort consisted of a random sample of 5,127 men and women aged 30 to 62, all residents of Framingham, Mass. Participants are reexamined every two years. . . . The present director is William P. Castelli, MD. *Lipid Research Clinics Study*. Started in the years 1972 to 1974, the study consists of a cohort of 8,000 individuals, about half of them women. It is a collaborative project of ten centers throughout the U.S. The principal purpose is to investigate the association between lipids and lipoproteins and subsequent cardiovascular disease. Trudy Bush, PhD, is conducting a follow-up study of the women in the original cohort. *Nurses' Health Study.* This study of 121,700 married female registered nurses, aged 30 to 55, was started in 1976 at Brigham and Women's Hospital, Boston, Mass. A questionnaire inquiring about the women's health and lifestyle practices is mailed every 2 years. The original questionnaire focused mainly on cardiovascular disease and cancer. . . . The director of the study is Frank Speizer, MD." *Contemporary Ob/Gyn* (November 1988), 115.

[18] Prevention and Management of Cardiovascular Risk in Women: 1989 Consensus Conference on Sex Hormones in Women, *Symposia Reporter,* 6, 11, 15-16; "Is ERT Cardioprotective?" *Menopause Management,* 7.

[19]*Contemporary Ob/Gyn* (November 1988), 108–23.

[20]Suggest that your physician read his latest journal articles about ERT and cardiovascular disease. The facts mentioned in this paragraph are taken from "How ERT Influences Cardiovascular Disease," *Contemporary Ob/Gyn* (November 1988), 108–23.

CHAPTER 11: IT'S NOT JUST YOUR IMAGINATION

[1]Shari Roan, "S.H.E. Shares Information on Risks of Hysterectomy," *Orange County Register* (September 2, 1987), E1.

[2]Burton Hillis, "The Man Next Door," *Better Homes and Gardens* (December 1989), 156.

CHAPTER 12: THE DOCTOR CONNECTION

[1]Ada P. Kahn and Linda Hughey Holt, *Midlife Health* (New York: Avon, 1987), 314–15.

CHAPTER 13: A PLACE FOR YOU

[1]As quoted in Betty Coble, *Women—Aware and Choosing* (Nashville: Broadman Press, 1975), 37.

CHAPTER 14: SETTING YOUR COURSE

[1]Richard Nelson Bolles, *What Color Is Your Parachute?* (Berkeley: Ten Speed Press). A new edition is published each year.

[2] Jim Conway, *Friendship: Skills for Having a Friend, Being a Friend* (Grand Rapids, MI: Zondervan Publishing House, 1989).

[3]Anne Morrow Lindbergh, *Gift from the Sea* (New York: Vintage, 1955, 1975), 96.

[4]Betty Coble, *Women—Aware and Choosing* (Nashville: Broadman Press, 1975).

CHAPTER 15: FOR HUSBANDS AND CHILDREN ONLY: UNDERSTANDING "MENO MAMA"

[1]My husband, Jim Conway, and I are the founders of Mid-Life Dimensions (Christian Living Resources, Inc.), which is a speaking, counseling, and writing ministry to help the mid-life generation with their specific issues. Books we have previously authored are listed in the Bibliography.

[2]See Galatians 6:1–2.

[3]Read Matthew 5:39–41.

Glossary

Amenorrhea. Absence of the menses (monthly period).

Arteriosclerosis. A chronic disease characterized by abnormal thickening and hardening of the arterial walls.

Atherosclerosis. A type of arteriosclerosis characterized by the deposition of fatty substances in the inner layer of the arteries.

Biopsy. The process of removing tissue from living patients for diagnosis.

Calcitonin. A "calcium-sparing" hormone released primarily by the thyroid gland. It acts to slow down the breakdown of bone.

Calcium. A metallic element found in nearly all living tissues. It gives bone most of its structural properties (99 percent of the body's calcium is in the bones) and is required for muscle contraction, blood clotting, and nerve impulse transmission.

Cardiovascular. Relating to the heart and the blood vessels or the circulation.

CAT (Computerized Axial Tomography) scan. A method of viewing cross sections of tissue or bone with X-rays.

-cele. A suffix denoting a swelling or hernia, as in *cystocele*.

Cervix. The narrow lower end of the uterus that extends into the vagina. (Pap smears are taken from the cervix.)

Cholesterol. A substance found especially in animal fats, blood, nerve tissue, and bile. If present in the blood in excessive amounts, it can be a factor in atherosclerosis.

Climacteric. A period in the life of a woman during the termination of the reproductive period; the time around menopause.

Collagen. A fibrous protein found in bone, connective tissue, cartilage, and skin.

Corpus luteum. Yellow tissue formed in the ovary in the site of a ruptured follicle that has discharged its ovum (egg). If the ovum is fertilized, this tissue secretes the hormone progesterone needed to maintain pregnancy.

Cortisone. An adrenal hormone that can harm bone. It also refers to a drug resembling the adrenal hormone, used in the treatment of various inflammatory diseases.

Cystocele. Hernia of the urinary bladder into the vagina.

D and C (dilation and curettage). A minor surgical procedure in which the cervical canal is enlarged to permit the scraping of the interior of the uterus for the removal of abnormal tissue or to obtain material for tissue diagnosis.

Diabetes. A disease that impairs the body's ability to use sugar.

Diuretic. A medication that increases the excretion of urine.

Dowager's hump. A protuberance of the upper back caused by painful collapsing of the vertebrae and outward curvature of the upper spine.

Dyspareunia. Pain during sexual intercourse.

-ectomy. Suffix meaning the removal of any organ or gland.

Endometrial. Relating to the inner lining of the uterine wall.

Endometrium. The lining of the uterus.

ERT. Estrogen replacement therapy.

Estrogen. The hormone responsible for the development and maintenance of female sex characteristics and reproductive function in women.

Fallopian tube. One of two tubes that branch from either side of the uterus; the tube through which the ovum (egg) passes from the ovary to the uterus.

Fibrocystic disease of the breast. A nonmalignant breast condition characterized by multiple small cysts and fibrous thickening of the breast tissue.

Fibroid. A nonmalignant tumor of the uterus; also called *leiomyomas* or *myomas*.

Follicle. One of the numerous depressions in the ovary, each containing an ovum (egg); sometimes called *Graafian follicle*.

Follicle stimulating hormone (FSH). Pituitary hormone that stimulates the growth and development of ovarian follicles.

FSH. See *follicle stimulating hormone*.

High density lipoproteins (HDL). Smallest and densest of lipoproteins that carry away excess cholesterol lining the arteries and that help to protect against atherosclerosis.

Hormone. A chemical substance formed in some organ of the body, as the pituitary, and carried in the blood to another part of the body where it has a specific effect.

Hormone replacement therapy (HRT). Treatment to restore

hormones lost by removal of the ovaries (as after a surgical menopause) or to correct a hormonal imbalance or deficiency (as can occur during a natural menopause).

HRT. See *hormone replacement therapy*.

Hyperplasia. An abnormal increase in the number of cells in a tissue or organ; often refers to buildup of endometrial tissue.

Hypertension. Abnormally high blood pressure.

Hypothalamus. A control center at the base of the brain that regulates body temperature, many metabolic processes, and certain emotional states.

Hysterectomy. Surgical removal of all or part of the uterus. A *total* or *complete hysterectomy* refers to surgical removal of both the uterus and cervix.

LDL. See *low-density lipo-proteins*.

LH. See *luteinizing hormone*.

Lipids. Fats that are insoluble in human blood plasma. Greasy to the touch, they are important constituents of living cells.

Lipoproteins. Any of a group of proteins combined with a lipid, found in blood plasma, egg yolk, brain tissue, etc.

Low density lipoproteins (LDL). Major lipoprotein for carrying cholesterol, which is essential for membrane synthesis. Excessive amounts of LDL cause deposits of plaque on arterial walls and increase the risk of coronary artery disease.

Luteinizing hormone (LH). Pituitary hormone that stimulates ovulation and the production of progesterone.

Malignant. Very dangerous or virulent; causing or likely to cause death. Often used to refer to a cancerous growth.

Mammography. An X-ray technique for the detection of breast tumors, cysts, or abnormal tissue changes before they can be seen or felt.

Menopause. The cessation of menses (monthly period).

Menses. The periodic flow of blood and sloughed-off tissue from the uterus, discharged through the genital tract.

Menstrual cycle. The time interval from the beginning of one menstrual period to the beginning of the next.

Metabolism. The chemical and physical processes continuously going on in the body, consisting of *anabolism*—the process by which food is changed into living tissues—and *catabolism*—the process by which living tissue is changed into energy and waste products.

Myomectomy. Surgical removal of a myoma (fibroid tumor) without removing the uterus.

Oophorectomy. Surgical removal of one or both ovaries.

Osteoblasts. Any cell that develops into bone or secretes substances producing bony tissues.

Osteoclasts. Any of the large cells in bone that absorb or break down bony tissue.

Osteoporosis. A bone disorder characterized by a reduction in overall bone mass accompanied by increased porosity and thinning of the bones, found chiefly in women who have passed menopause or men and women over age 65.

Ovary. The female sex gland that produces eggs (ova).

Ovulation. The release of an ovum (egg) from the ovarian follicle.

Ovum (plural, ova). The female sex cell produced by the ovaries.

Pap smear. Common name for Papanicolaou smear. A method whereby cells from the vagina are microscopically examined for any abnormal changes. Used as a screening method for cervical cancer.

Pituitary gland. A small oval organ at the base of the brain; it produces many important hormones and has been called the "master gland."

Plaque. A deposit of fatty or fibrous material in a blood vessel wall.

Plasma. Fluid part of the blood.

Postmenopausal. After the menopause.

Precursor. A forerunner or "building block."

Premenopausal. Before the menopause.

Progesterone. The hormone produced by the ovary during the second half of the menstrual cycle. It acts to prepare the uterus for pregnancy.

Prolapse. A falling down of an organ because of inadequate muscular support, as in a prolapsed uterus.

Receptor. A tiny area on the surface of cells or membranes at which specific substances "fit" (like a lock and key) and exert their effects.

Rectocele. A bulging of the rectal wall into the vaginal canal.

Salpingectomy. Surgical removal of a fallopian tube.

Salpingo-. Combining form meaning tube, usually refers to fallopian tube.

Saturated fats. Fats of animal origin including meat fat, butter, whole milk, cream, and cheeses made from whole milk or cream. Unsaturated fats may become saturated through hydrogenation and are used in many processed foods. Some vegetable fats, such as coconut oil, palm oil, and cocoa butter are also saturated. Saturated fats tend to raise the cholesterol level.

Surgical menopause. A premature menopause brought on by surgical removal of the ovaries before the woman has experienced a natural menopause.

Triglycerides. Neutral fatty substances found in the blood and fat cells.

Uterus. The womb; the hollow muscular organ in which the impregnated ovum is developed into a baby.

Vagina. The canal extending from the uterus to the outside.

Vasomotor. Nerves that regulate the size in diameter of blood vessels.

BIBLIOGRAPHY

MENOPAUSE AND MENOPAUSE CONCERNS

Beard, Mary K. and Lindsay Curtis. *Menopause and the Years Ahead*. Tucson: Fisher Books, 1988.

Budoff, Penny Wise. *No More Hot Flashes and Other Good News*. New York: Warner, 1984.

Cooper, Kenneth H. *Preventing Osteoporosis*. New York: Bantam, 1989.

McIlwain, Harris H., Debra Fulghum Bruce, Joel C. Silverfield, and Michael C. Burnette. *Osteoporosis: Prevention, Management, Treatment*. New York: John Wiley & Sons, 1988.

Nachtigall, Lila, and Joan Rattner Heilman. *Estrogen: The Facts Can Change Your Life*. Los Angeles: The Body Press, division of Price Stern Sloan, 1986.

Notelovitz, Morris, and Marsha Ware. *Stand Tall! The Informed Woman's Guide to Preventing Osteoporosis*. Gainesville, Fla: Triad, 1982.

Schoenfeld, Orene V., and Beverly Bush Smith. *Change for the Better*. Old Tappan, NJ: Revell, 1986.

GENERAL HEALTH

Kahn, Ada P. and Linda Hughey Holt. *Midlife Health*. New York: Avon Books, 1987.

Sneed, Dr. Sharon and Sneed, Dr. David. *Prime Time: A Complete Health Guide for Women 35 to 65*. Dallas: Word Publishing, 1989.

SEXUAL GUIDANCE

Clifford and Joyce Penner. *The Gift of Sex*. Waco, Tex.: Word, 1981.

Wheat, Ed, M.D., and Gaye Wheat. *Intended for Pleasure*. Old Tappan, NJ: Revell, 1977.

PERSONAL GROWTH, MARRIAGE, AND FAMILY

Bolles, Richard Nelson. *What Color Is Your Parachute?* Berkeley: Ten Speed Press, a new edition is published each year.

Coble, Betty. *Woman—Aware and Choosing*. Nashville: Broadman, 1975.

Conway, Jim. *Friendship: Skills for Having a Friend, Being a Friend*. Grand Rapids: Zondervan, 1989.

Conway, Jim. *Men in Mid-Life Crisis*. Elgin, Ill.: David C. Cook, 1978.

Conway, Jim and Sally Conway. *Women in Mid-Life Crisis*. Wheaton, Ill.: Tyndale House, 1983.

Conway, Jim and Sally. *Your Marriage Can Survive Mid-Life Crisis: Ten Keys to an Intimate Marriage*. Nashville: Thomas Nelson, 1987.

Conway, Sally. *Your Husband's Mid-Life Crisis*. Elgin, Ill.: David C. Cook, 1980.

Dobson, James. *What Wives Wish Their Husbands Knew about Women*. Wheaton, Ill.: Tyndale House, 1975.

Lindbergh, Anne Morrow. *Gift from the Sea*. New York: Vintage, 1955, 1975.

Lush, Jean. *Emotional Phases of a Woman's Life*. Old Tappan, NJ: Revell, 1987.

Sanders, Becki Conway and Conway, Jim and Sally. *What God Gives When Life Takes*. Downers Grove, Ill.: InterVarsity, 1989.

INDEX

NATIONAL STUDY OF MENOPAUSE

NOTE: This is a sample questionnaire for your information only. Please do *not* complete and send in.

If you have experienced menopause (naturally or surgically), or:

If you think you are having premenopausal symptoms, PLEASE FILL OUT THIS QUESTIONNAIRE AND MAIL TO: Sally Conway.

DEFINITIONS FOR THIS SURVEY:

Menopause–complete cessation of menstruation, an exact point in time

Premenopause–the years immediately prior to menopause

Postmenopause–all time after menopause

Symptoms–physical and emotional conditions or signs relating to menopause

Hormone Replacement Therapy (HRT)–estrogen and/or progesterone prescribed to compensate for the natural decline in the body; may be in the form of pills, injections, dermal patches, etc.

Today's Date _____ Your Birth Year _____ Zip Code _____

1. **Please circle the letter of the category that fits you:**
   a. I **have not** yet experienced menopause, but I believe I am having menopausal symptoms.

b. I **have not** yet experienced menopause, but I was having symptoms and I am on hormone replacement therapy.

c. I **have** experienced menopause, and I am on hormone replacement therapy.

d. I **have** experienced menopause, and I am not presently on hormone replacement therapy, but I have had hormone replacement therapy.

e. I **have** experienced menopause, and I have never had hormone replacement therapy.

IF YOU **HAVE NOT** YET EXPERIENCED MENOPAUSE, SKIP TO QUESTION #7
IF YOU **HAVE** EXPERIENCED MENOPAUSE, GO TO QUESTION #2

2. Was your menopause natural or surgical ("surgical" means a complete hysterectomy, including removal of both ovaries)? Natural _____ Surgical _____ At what age did this occur? _____

3. Approximately how many years did you experience premenopausal symptoms?   _____ years

4. Have you experienced postmenopausal symptoms? Yes _____   No _____

    (If No, skip to question #7.)

5. Are you still experiencing postmenopausal symptoms? Yes _____   No _____

(If Yes, skip to question #7. If No, answer question #6.)

6. Approximately how many years did you experience postmenopausal symptoms?   _____ years

7. **Please comment on the type and severity of your symptoms**—both pre- and post-, with or without hormone replacement therapy. (Some symptoms, such as "irritable," should be compared to your normal state prior to the onset of menopausal symptoms. For instance, in earlier years you may have experienced a certain degree of irritability at times, but

during the menopausal years you may have a great deal more irritability.)

		None (0)	Slight (1)	Moderate (2)	Extreme (3)
a.	Hot flashes	0	1	2	3
b.	Nervousness ("jumpy")	0	1	2	3
c.	Irritability (grumpy)	0	1	2	3
d.	Crying spells	0	1	2	3
e.	Impatience	0	1	2	3
f.	Anger	0	1	2	3
g.	Depression	0	1	2	3
h.	Anxiety	0	1	2	3
i.	Strange skin sensations	0	1	2	3
j.	Dry skin	0	1	2	3
k.	Vaginal dryness	0	1	2	3
l.	Heart palpitations	0	1	2	3
m.	Unhealthy hair	0	1	2	3
n.	Unhealthy nails	0	1	2	3
o.	Loss of sexual desire	0	1	2	3
p.	Forgetfulness	0	1	2	3
q.	Sleep problems	0	1	2	3
r.	Low self-esteem	0	1	2	3
s.	Jealousy	0	1	2	3
t.	Suspicion	0	1	2	3
u.	Insecurity	0	1	2	3
v.	Urinary incontinence	0	1	2	3
w.	Painful joints	0	1	2	3
x.	Thoughts of suicide	0	1	2	3
y.	Fatalistic view of life	0	1	2	3
z.	Excessive bleeding	0	1	2	3

Other behaviors or feelings _____

8. Now go back over the previous list of symptoms and "star" the four symptoms which cause, or caused, you the **most distress**. (NOTE: A symptom that is, or was, very severe may not have

distressed you as much as a less severe symptom. For example, extreme hot flashes may not have bothered you as much as a slight problem with anxiety.)

9. Circle the following which have been helpful to you in relieving your **physical symptoms**.

		Does not apply	No help	Slightly helpful	Moderately helpful	Great help
		(0)	(1)	(2)	(3)	(4)
a.	Hormone therapy (estrogen replacement)	0	1	2	3	4
b.	Other prescriptions, such as	0	1	2	3	4
c.	Over-the-counter preparations, such as	0	1	2	3	4
d.	The passing of time	0	1	2	3	4
e.	Other helps, such as	0	1	2	3	4

10. Which of the following have been helpful to you in relieving your **emotional** symptoms?

		Does not apply	No help	Slightly helpful	Moderately helpful	Great help
		(0)	(1)	(2)	(3)	(4)
a.	Your husband's care	0	1	2	3	4
b.	Your child or children	0	1	2	3	4
c.	Your mother	0	1	2	3	4
d.	Another older relative or older friend	0	1	2	3	4
e.	Friend(s) your age	0	1	2	3	4
f.	Your doctor (M.D.)	0	1	2	3	4

    (1)   How many doctors have you seen regarding menopause? _____

		Does not apply	No help	Slightly helpful	Moderately helpful	Great help
		(0)	(1)	(2)	(3)	(4)

(2)   How many doctors have been helpful? _____

		Does not apply	No help	Slightly helpful	Moderately helpful	Great help
g.	Another professional	0	1	2	3	4
	What profession? _____					
h.	Reading a book(s) about menopause	0	1	2	3	4
	Titles _____					
i.	Other self-help books	0	1	2	3	4
	Titles or kinds _____					
j.	Magazine articles	0	1	2	3	4
	Names of magazines _____					
k.	Television and/or radio programs about menopause	0	1	2	3	4
l.	Worship services	0	1	2	3	4
m.	Attending a class	0	1	2	3	4
	What kind of class? _____					
n.	A small care group	0	1	2	3	4
o.	Personal prayer	0	1	2	3	4
p.	Reading the Bible	0	1	2	3	4
q.	Keeping busy	0	1	2	3	4
r.	Resting more	0	1	2	3	4
s.	Exercise	0	1	2	3	4
t.	A new hobby or interest	0	1	2	3	4
u.	More involvement in a career	0	1	2	3	4

Other help _____

11. How did or does menopause affect your relationships?

		No Effect	Very Negatively	Somewhat Negatively	Somewhat Positively	Very Positively
		(0)	(1)	(2)	(3)	(4)
a.	Marriage	0	1	2	3	4
b.	Children	0	1	2	3	4
c.	Parents	0	1	2	3	4
d.	Friends	0	1	2	3	4
e.	Work colleagues	0	1	2	3	4

Other comments _____

12. What else would you like to tell me that you have found **difficult** during menopause? (If you need more space, use a separate sheet of paper.)

13. What else would you like to tell me that you have found **helpful during menopause?** (If you need more space, use a separate piece of paper.)